ALLE · ZEIT · WACH · 1842

Wolfgang Jelkmann
Andreas J. Gross (Eds.)

Erythropoietin

Foreword by P. Mary Cotes

With 55 Figures and 14 Tables

Springer-Verlag Berlin Heidelberg New York
London Paris Tokyo Hong Kong

Professor Dr. med. WOLFGANG JELKMANN
Dr. med. ANDREAS J. GROSS

Physiologisches Institut
Medizinische Universität zu Lübeck
Ratzeburger Allee 160
2400 Lübeck 1
Federal Republic of Germany

ISBN-13: 978-3-642-83747-0 e-ISBN-13: 978-3-642-83745-6
DOI: 10.1007/978-3-642-83745-6

Library of Congress Cataloging-in-Publication Data
Erythropoietin / Wolfgang Jelkmann, Andreas J. Gross (eds.). p. cm. Includes bibliographies and index. ISBN 0-387-50955-0 (U.S.: alk. paper) 1. Erythropoietin-Physiological effect. 2. Erythropoietin-Therapeutic use. 3. Anemia-Chemotherapy. I. Jelkmann, Wolfgang, 1949. II. Gross, Andreas J., 1958. [DNLM: 1. Anemia-drug therapy. 2. Erythropoiesis. 3. Erythropoietin-physiology. 4. Erythropoietin-therapeutic use. WH 150 E735] QP96.E784 1989 612.1'11-dc20 DNLM/DLC

Softcover reprint of the hardcover 1st edition 1989

Typesetting and printing: Meininger GmbH, Neustadt
Bookbinding: Schäffer GmbH & Co. KG, Grünstadt
2127/3145-543210 – Printed on acid-free paper

Foreword

Recent developments in recombinant DNA technology have led to the large-scale production of human erythropoietin and to the demonstration that it is effective in the treatment of renal and possibly some other anaemias. This has lent a new impetus to studies of the pathophysiology and pharmacology of the hormone which is reflected in this report of the proceedings of a meeting held in Lübeck in June 1988.

In 15 papers, all from European centres, the broad topics covered are erythropoietin's physiology and chemistry, the pathophysiology of erythropoiesis and the use of erythropoietin in the treatment of anaemia. Several of the papers include up-to-date reviews of the literature. The field is now expanding rapidly, and this volume, though not comprehensive, usefully points up many areas of recent understanding as well as others of continuing uncertainty. Overall, it contains material likely to be of interest to biochemists and experimental haematologists as well as to pharmacologists, clinical haematologists and nephrologists.

P. Mary Cotes

List of Contents

List of Contributors

BALCKE, P.
I. Medizinische Universitätsklinik, Lazarettgasse 14, 1090 Wien, Austria

BARIETY, J.
INSERM U 28, Hôpital Broussais, 96, rue Didot, 75014 Paris, France

BATTERSBY, R. V.
IBR Bioanalytical Centre, Feodor-Lynen-Strasse 5, 3000 Hannover 61, Federal Republic of Germany

BRUNEVAL, P.
INSERM U 28, Hôpital Broussais, 96, rue Didot, 75014 Paris, France

CAMILLERI, J.-P.
INSERM U 28, Hôpital Broussais, 96, rue Didot, 75014 Paris, France

CAROZZI, S.
Unit of Nephrology and Dialysis, St. Paul's Hospital, Monoblocco Valloria, 17100 Savona, Italy

CLEMONS, G. K.
Lawrence Berkeley Laboratory, University of California, 1 Cyclotron Road, Berkeley, CA 94720, USA

COTES, P. M.
Clinical Research Centre, Watford Road, Harrow, Middlesex HA1 3UJ, United Kingdom

DJUKANOVIĆ, L.
Institute for Kidney Diseases, KBC Zvezdara, 11001 Beograd, Yugoslavia

GANSER, A.
Abteilung für Hämatologie, Zentrum der Inneren Medizin, Klinikum der J. W. Goethe-Universität, Theodor-Stern-Kai 7, 6000 Frankfurt/M 70, Federal Republic of Germany

GEISSLER, K.
I. Medizinische Universitätsklinik, Lazarettgasse 14, 1090 Wien, Austria

GRAF, H.
II. Medizinische Universitätsklinik, Garnisongasse 13, 1090 Wien, Austria

GROSS, A. J.
Physiologisches Institut, Medizinische Universität zu Lübeck, Ratzeburger Allee 160, 2400 Lübeck 1, Federal Republic of Germany

GRÜTZMACHER, P.
Abteilung für Nephrologie, Zentrum der Inneren Medizin, Klinikum der J. W. Goethe-Universität, Theodor-Stern-Kai 7, 6000 Frankfurt/M 70, Federal Republic of Germany

HÅGÅ, P.
Departments of Pathology and Pediatrics, Oslo Kommune, Ulleval Sykehus, Kirkeveien 166, 0407 Oslo 4, Norway

HALVORSEN, S.
Departments of Pathology and Pediatrics, Oslo Kommune, Ulleval Sykehus, Kirkeveien 166, 0407 Oslo 4, Norway

HEIDLAND, A.
Abteilung für Nephrologie, Medizinische Universitätsklinik, Josef-Schneider-Strasse 2, 8700 Würzburg, Federal Republic of Germany

HELLEBOSTAD, M.
Departments of Pathology and Pediatrics, Oslo Kommune, Ulleval Sykehus, Kirkeveien 166, 0407 Oslo 4, Norway

HINTERBERGER, W.
I. Medizinische Universitätsklinik, Lazarettgasse 14, 1090 Wien, Austria

HOELZER, D.
Abteilung für Hämatologie, Zentrum der Inneren Medizin, Klinikum der J. W. Goethe-Universität, Theodor-Stern-Kai 7, 6000 Frankfurt/M 70, Federal Republic of Germany

HOLLOWAY, C. J.
IBR Bioanalytical Centre, Feodor-Lynen-Strasse 5, 3000 Hannover 61, Federal Republic of Germany

HOLTER, P.
Departments of Pathology and Pediatrics, Oslo Kommune, Ulleval Sykehus, Kirkeveien 166, 0407 Oslo 4, Norway

JELKMANN, W.
Physiologisches Institut, Medizinische Universität zu Lübeck, Ratzeburger Allee 160, 2400 Lübeck 1, Federal Republic of Germany

JOHANNSEN, H.
Physiologisches Institut, Medizinische Universität zu Lübeck, Ratzeburger Allee 160, 2400 Lübeck 1, Federal Republic of Germany

LACOMBE, C.
INSERM U 152 and CNRS UA 628, Hôpital Cochin, 27, rue du Faubourg Saint-Jacques, 75014 Paris, France

LAMPERI, S.
St. Martin's Hospital, Viale Benedetto XV-10, 16132 Genova, Italy

LAPPIN, T. R. J.
Eastern Health & Social Services Board, Royal Victoria Hospital, Belfast BT12 6BA, Northern Ireland

MAXWELL, A. P.
Eastern Health & Social Services Board, Royal Victoria Hospital, Belfast BT12 6BA, Northern Ireland

MEBERG, A.
Departments of Pathology and Pediatrics, Oslo Kommune, Ulleval Sykehus, Kirkeveien 166, 0407 Oslo 4, Norway

MAYER, G.
II. Medizinische Universitätsklinik, Garnisongasse 13, 1090 Wien, Austria

NASINI, M. G.
St. Martin's Hospital, Viale Benedetto XV-10, 16132 Genova, Italy

PAGEL, H.
Physiologisches Institut, Medizinische Universität zu Lübeck, Ratzeburger Allee 160, 2400 Lübeck 1, Federal Republic of Germany

PAVLOVIĆ-KENTERA, V.
Institute for Medical Research, Bul. JNA 10, P. O. Box 721, 11001 Beograd, Yugoslavia

RICH, I. N.
Abteilung für Transfusionsmedizin der Universität Ulm, Oberer Eselsberg 10, 7900 Ulm/Donau, Federal Republic of Germany

SALZMANN, J.-L.
INSERM U 28, Hôpital Broussais, 96, rue Didot, 75014 Paris, France

SANENGEN, T.
Departments of Pathology and Pediatrics, Oslo Kommune, Ulleval Sykehus, Kirkeveien 166, 0407 Oslo 4, Norway

SCHAEFER, R. M.
Abteilung für Nephrologie, Medizinische Universitätsklinik, Josef-Schneider-Strasse 2, 8700 Würzburg, Federal Republic of Germany

W. SCHOEPPE
Abteilung für Nephrologie, Zentrum der Inneren Medizin, Klinikum der J. W. Goethe-Universität, Theodor-Stern-Kai 7, 6000 Frankfurt/M 70, Federal Republic of Germany

DA SILVA, J.-L.
INSERM U 28, Hôpital Broussais, 96, rue Didot, 75014 Paris, France

STOCKENHUBER, F.
I. Medizinische Universitätsklinik, Lazarettgasse 14, 1090 Wien, Austria

TAMBOURIN, P.
INSERM U 152 and CNRS UA 628, Hôpital Cochin, 27, rue du Faubourg Saint-Jacques, 75014 Paris, France

VARET, B.
INSERM U 152 and CNRS UA 628, Hôpital Cochin, 27, rue du Faubourg Saint-Jacques, 75014 Paris, France

WEISS, C.
Physiologisches Institut, Universität zu Lübeck, Ratzeburger Allee 160, 2400 Lübeck 1, Federal Republic of Germany

Introduction: Advances in Erythropoietin Research

W. JELKMANN and A. J. GROSS

New blood cells are permanently generated from stem cells in the hemopoietically active bone marrow. Pluripotent hematopoietic stem cells have the capacity to self-replicate and to produce progeny committed to any of the different lineages of blood cells. Little is known about the mechanisms which control the differentiation of the pluripotent stem cells. The glycoprotein hormone erythropoietin stimulates the proliferation and differentiation of progenitor cells committed to the erythrocytic lineage (Fig. 1).

The French anatomist Viault [34] first reported that erythropoiesis is acutely stimulated following exposure to low O_2 pressure at altitude. When Viault travelled to Morococha (4400 m) in Peru, the number of erythrocytes in his blood increased from 5 to 8 millions per microliter within 23 days. More recently, physical training of athletes at altitude has been applied to improve their endurance performance.

The existence of a humoral factor *("hémopoïétine")* controlling erythropoiesis was first proposed by Carnot and Deflandre [4]. When these investigators injected

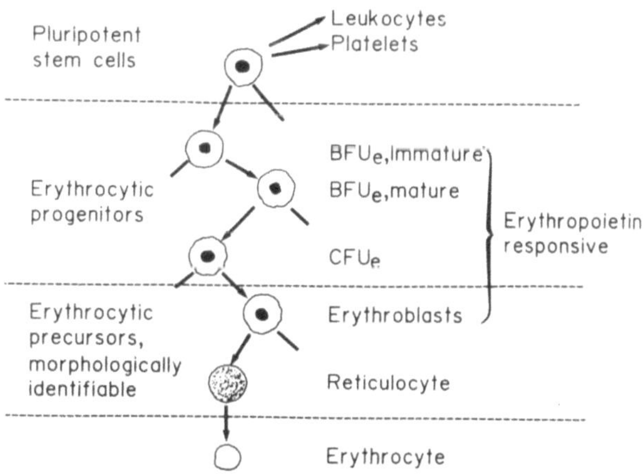

Fig. 1. The major differentiation steps in bone marrow erythropoiesis. Erythropoietin stimulates the proliferation and differentiation of the erythrocytic progenitors (*BFU*$_e$ burst-forming unit-erythroid; *CFU*$_e$, colony-forming unit-erythroid). The CFU$_e$ is the main target cell of erythropoietin. Reproduced from [20]

serum from (slightly) anemic rabbits into normal animals the red blood cell number increased in the recipients within 2 days. Subsequent studies failed, however, to confirm this rapid and strong response. In addition, it has been previously shown that erythropoietin induces reticulocytosis only after a lag of 2–4 days [9, 28].

The concept of the hormonal control of erythropoiesis was not generally accepted (for references, see [11, 20]), until Ruhenstroth-Bauer [31] and Reissmann [30] reported their parabiosis studies. In parabiotic animals, the formation of reticulocytes increased in both partners when anemia or hypoxemia was induced in one of them. Erslev then carried out a re-investigation of the experiment of Carnot and Deflandre [9]. He observed a reticulocytosis and – in the long term – an increase in hematocrit in rabbits repeatedly infused with large volumes (100–200 ml) of plasma from severely anemic donor rabbits. This study provided real evidence for the existence of a humoral erythropoiesis-stimulating factor. Erslev predicted that "isolation and purification of this factor would provide an agent useful in the treatment of conditions associated with erythropoietic depression, such as chronic infection and chronic renal disease".

Tissue hypoxia is the major stimulus for the synthesis of erythropoietin. In severe anemia or hypoxemia erythropoietin levels may reach 10 000 mU/ml plasma, compared to a normal value of about 10 mU/ml (for a definition of the erythropoietin unit, see [1]). The important role of the kidneys in the elaboration of erythropoietin was noted by Jacobson et al., who found that bilateral nephrectomy abolishes the erythropoietin response in anemic rats [19]. Kuratowska et al. [23] and Fisher and Birdwell [13] first reported erythropoietin production by isolated kidneys perfused with blood. For some years, it was believed that renal cells could not synthetize erythropoietin directly, but produced an enzyme capable of splitting a proerythropoietin produced by the liver [17]. However, this concept became less likely when Erslev demonstrated erythropoietin in the serum-free perfusate of isolated kidneys [10]. Erythropoietin was later extracted from the cortex of hypoxic kidneys flushed free of blood [21]. Final proof of a direct renal origin of the hormone was provided with the demonstration of erythropoietin mRNA in the kidney [2, 3, 33]. Most likely, peritubular capillary cells in the kidney cortex are the site of the production of erythropoietin [22, 24].

Erythropoietin mRNA was also demonstrated in the liver [2, 3]. The liver is regarded as the main extrarenal site of the production of erythropoietin [14]. Recent studies in human hepatoma cell cultures have provided some evidence that an intracellular heme protein is involved in the mechanism by which hypoxia stimulates the synthesis of erythropoietin [16].

The purification of erythropoietin from human urine [27] certainly has been one of the most important steps in erythropoietin research. The availability of pure erythropoietin has enabled investigators to develop reliable radioimmunoassays for the hormone [5, 15], which are increasingly used instead of the long-established bioassays in exhypoxic [6] or hypertransfused polycythemic mice. The partial identification of the amino acid sequence of purified human urinary erythropoietin was the initial step in the isolation and the in vitro expression of the human erythropoietin gene in cultured mammalian cells [18, 25, 26]. Chinese hamster ovary cells (CHO cells) are presently used in the industrial production of recombinant human erythropoietin for clinical purposes. This recombinant human erythropoietin – like the natural hormone – is a posttranslationally modified glycoprotein and exhibits similar biological effects [7, 8, 29, 32].

The availability of recombinant human erythropoietin has provided a new tool in the treatment of severe anemia. Winearls et al. [35] and Eschbach et al. [12] first reported that the replacement therapy with erythropoietin can restore the hematocrit to normal in patients with end-stage renal failure, thus preventing the need for transfusions with their risk of infections and iron overload.

In view of the increasing importance of erythropoietin as a therapeutic agent, a meeting on the pathophysiology and pharmacology of the hormone was held in Lübeck in June, 1988. Participants of this meeting have contributed to the present monograph.

References

1. Annable L, Cotes PM, Mussett MV (1972) The second international reference preparation of erythropoietin, human, urinary, for bioassay. Bull WHO 47: 99–112
2. Beru N, McDonald J, Lacombe C, Goldwasser E (1986) Expression of the erythropoietin gene. Mol Cell Biol 6: 2571–2575
3. Bondurant MC, Koury MJ (1986) Anemia induces accumulation of erythropoietin mRNA in the kidney and liver. Mol Cell Biol 6: 2731–2733
4. Carnot P, Deflandre C (1906) Sur l'activité hémopoïétique des différents organes au cours de la régénération du sang. CR Acad Sci Paris 143: 432–435
5. Cotes PM (1982) Immunoreactive erythropoietin in serum. Br J Haematol 50: 427–438
6. Cotes PM, Bangham DR (1961) Bio-assay of erythropoietin in mice made polycythaemic by exposure to air at a reduced pressure. Nature 191: 1065–1067
7. Davis JM, Arakawa T, Strickland TW, Yphantis DA (1987) Characterization of recombinant human erythropoietin produced in Chinese hamster ovary cells. Biochemistry 26: 2633–2638
8. Egrie JC, Strickland TW, Lane J, Aoki K, Cohen AM, Smalling R, Trail G, Lin FK, Browne JK, Hines DK (1986) Characterization and biological effects of recombinant human erythropoietin. Immunobiology 172: 213–224
9. Erslev A (1953) Humoral regulation of red cell production. Blood 8: 349–357
10. Erslev AJ (1974) In vitro production of erythropoietin by kidneys perfused with a serum-free solution. Blood 44: 77–85
11. Erslev AJ (1980) Blood and mountains. In: Wintrobe MM (ed) Blood, pure and eloquent. McGraw-Hill, New York, pp 257–280
12. Eschbach JW, Egrie JC, Downing MR, Browne JK, Adamson JW (1987) Correction of the anemia of end-stage renal disease with recombinant human erythropoietin. N Engl J Med 316: 73–78
13. Fisher JW, Birdwell BJ (1961) The production of an erythropoietic factor by the in situ perfused kidney. Acta Haematol 26: 224–232
14. Fried W (1972) The liver as a source of extrarenal erythropoietin production. Blood 40: 671–677
15. Garcia JF, Sherwood J, Goldwasser E (1979) Radioimmunoassay of erythropoietin. Blood Cells 5: 405–419

16. Goldberg MA, Dunning SP, Bunn HF (1988) Regulation of the erythropoietin gene: Evidence that the oxygen sensor is a heme protein. Science 242: 1412–1415
17. Gordon AS, Cooper GW, Zanjani ED (1967) The kidney and erythropoiesis. Semin Hematol 4: 337–358
18. Jacobs K, Shoemaker C, Rudersdorf R, Neill SD, Kaufman RJ, Mufson A, Seehra J, Jones SS, Hewick R, Fritsch EF, Kawakita M, Shimizu T, Miyake T (1985) Isolation and characterization of genomic and cDNA clones of human erythropoietin. Nature 313: 806–810
19. Jacobson LO, Goldwasser E, Fried W, Plzak L (1957) Role of the kidney in erythropoiesis. Nature 179: 633–634
20. Jelkmann W (1986) Erythropoietin research, 80 years after the initial studies by Carnot and Deflandre. Respir Physiol 63: 257–266
21. Jelkmann W, Bauer C (1981) Demonstration of high levels of erythropoietin in rat kidneys following hypoxic hypoxia. Pflügers Arch 392: 34–39
22. Koury ST, Bondurant MC, Koury MJ (1988) Localization of erythropoietin synthesizing cells in murine kidneys by in situ hybridization. Blood 71: 524–527
23. Kuratowska Z, Lewartowski B, Michalak E (1961) Studies on the production of erythropoietin by isolated perfused organs. Blood 18: 527–534
24. Lacombe C, DaSilva JL, Bruneval P, Fournier JG, Wendling F, Casadevall N, Camilleri JP, Bariety J, Varet B, Tambourin P (1988) Peritubular cells are the site of erythropoietin synthesis in the murine hypoxic kidney. J Clin Invest 81: 620–623
25. Lai PH, Everett R, Wang FF, Arakawa T, Goldwasser E (1986) Structural characterization of human erythropoietin. J Biol Chem 261: 3116–3121
26. Lin FK, Suggs S, Lin CH, Browne JK, Smalling R, Egrie JC, Chen KK, Fox GM, Martin F, Stabinsky Z, Badrawi SM, Lai PH, Goldwasser E (1985) Cloning and expression of the human erythropoietin gene. Proc Natl Acad Sci USA 82: 7580–7584
27. Miyake T, Kung CKH, Goldwasser E (1977) Purification of human erythropoietin. J Biol Chem 252: 5558–5564
28. Papayannopoulou T, Finch CA (1972) On the in vivo action of erythropoietin: a quantitative analysis. J Clin Invest 51: 1179–1185
29. Recny MA, Scoble HA, Kim Y (1987) Structural characterization of natural human urinary and recombinant DNA-derived erythropoietin. J Biol Chem 262: 17156–17163
30. Reissmann KR (1950) Studies on the mechanism of erythropoietic stimulation in parabiotic rats during hypoxia. Blood 5: 372–380
31. Ruhenstroth-Bauer G (1950) Versuche zum Nachweis eines spezifischen erythropoetischen Hormons. Arch Exp Pathol Pharmakol 211: 32–56
32. Sasaki H, Bothner B, Dell A, Fukuda M (1987) Carbohydrate structure of erythropoietin expressed in Chinese hamster ovary cells by a human erythropoietin cDNA. J Biol Chem 262: 12059–12076
33. Schuster SJ, Wilson JH, Erslev AJ, Caro J (1987) Physiologic regulation and tissue localization of renal erythropoietin messenger RNA. Blood 70: 316–318
34. Viault F (1980) Sur l'augmentation considérable du nombre des globules rouges dans le sang chez les habitants des hauts plateaux de l'Amérique du Sud. CR Acad Sci Paris 111: 917–918
35. Winearls CG, Oliver DO, Pippard MJ, Reid C, Downing MR, Cotes PM (1986) Effect of human erythropoietin derived from recombinant DNA on the anaemia of patients maintained by chronic haemodialysis. Lancet ii: 1175–1178

Chemistry and Physiology

Chemistry and Assays of Erythropoietin

T. R. J. LAPPIN and A. P. MAXWELL

Chemistry of Erythropoietin

Introduction

The current therapeutic use of erythropoietin (Epo) represents the culmination of a difficult struggle to isolate, purify and characterise the hormone. Epo is the principal regulatory hormone of the circulating red cell mass [1, 2] and is normally present in minute concentrations in serum at 15–30 milliunits/ml, or approximately $10^{-11} M$ [3–5]. The study of Epo has been hampered for many years by its extreme scarcity and the lack of a convenient assay.

Epo is a glycoprotein with an Mr of 30400 as determined by sedimentation equilibrium experiments [6]. The Epo molecule is hydrophobic, withstands heating to 80 °C and retains biological activity after exposure to: (1) extremes of pH from 3.5 to 10.0; (2) a variety of solvents; and (3) certain chaotropic agents [7–11].

The monumental task of purifying Epo was reported in 1977 by Miyake et al. [12]. Starting from 2550 l of urine collected from patients with aplastic anaemia, they produced a small quantity of purified Epo with a specific activity of 70400 U/mg of protein. This represented an overall purification factor of 930 and the purified material was the starting point for attempts to clone the Epo gene.

Isolation and Expression of the Human Erythropoietin Gene

The absence of a source of human Epo messenger RNA hindered attempts to isolate the erythropoietin gene. Two separate strategies were adopted to overcome this difficulty. Lin et al. [13] isolated the gene directly from a genomic DNA library whilst Jacobs et al. [14] screened a fetal liver cDNA library recovering a clone with the intact gene. Both groups working independently achieved expression of the Epo gene in suitable vectors and published their findings in 1985. This landmark in erythropoietin research paved the way for unlimited quantities of recombinant human erythropoietin (rHu Epo) to be produced. Further detailed chemical analysis of the molecule was then possible and human clinical trials began in 1985.

The cloning strategies both involved using mixtures of oligonucleotide probes to search DNA libraries. The amino acid sequence data derived from limited tryptic digestion of human urinary Epo (U-Epo) provided the basic information required to direct the synthesis of the oligonucleotide probes. The degeneracy of the genetic code meant that many oligonucleotide probes were needed to ensure that one probe would correctly locate Epo messenger RNA in a DNA library.

Lai et al. [15] isolated and sequenced tryptic digest fragments of Epo using a gas-phase microsequencer. Lin et al. [13] selected a hexapeptide and a heptapeptide with low codon degeneracy for synthesis of the corresponding 17-mer and 20-mer oligodeoxynucleotides. Each of the two probe mixtures synthesized contained a pool of 128 oligonucleotide sequences, and these permitted the rapid isolation of the Epo gene from a human genomic library. Chinese hamster ovary (CHO) cells were transformed with an expression vector containing the Epo gene and biologically active rHu Epo was recovered.

Jacobs et al. [14] also used tryptic fragment data to prepare four pools of highly degenerate oligonucleotide probes in order to isolate the Epo gene from a bacteriophage library of human genomic DNA. They demonstrated that human fetal liver is a source of Epo mRNA for complementary DNA cloning, using a 95-nucleotide single-stranded probe prepared from an M13 cloning vector which contained a fragment of the Epo gene. The fetal liver cDNA library was screened and an Epo cDNA clone was identified. COS cells were transfected with the Epo clone and transient expression of the Epo gene was achieved.

The amino acid sequence deduced from the nucleotide sequence agrees precisely with the protein sequence data, confirming that the isolated cDNA encodes human Epo [14]. Analysis of the DNA sequence of Epo does not support the suggestion [16] that renin substrate may be the Epo precursor [14].

The Epo gene is located on the long arm of chromosome 7 [17, 18] and exists as a single copy per haploid human genome [13, 14]. The gene, which contains five exons and four introns, encodes a 193 residue polypeptide, the first 27 amino acids of which represent a leader sequence which is cleaved on secretion.

Primary Protein Structure

The primary structure of human Epo, based on protein sequence analysis [15], is shown in Fig. 1. The 166-residue polypeptide has a calculated Mr of 18400 for the protein moiety. Subsequent analysis of the C-terminus by peptide mapping and fast atom bombardment mass spectrometry (FABMS) indicated that the arginyl residue, assumed to be present in the C-terminal position, is missing from both human U-Epo and rHu Epo [19]. The term des-arginine 166 erythropoietin has been used to distinguish the truncated molecule from the structure originally deduced from the genomic [13], cDNA [14] and protein sequences [15].

The 166-amino-acid molecule contains 39 charged residues of which 21 are basic and 18 are acidic. No charged residues are present in residues 77–88, suggesting that this region of the molecule is internal. Both the N-terminal and C-

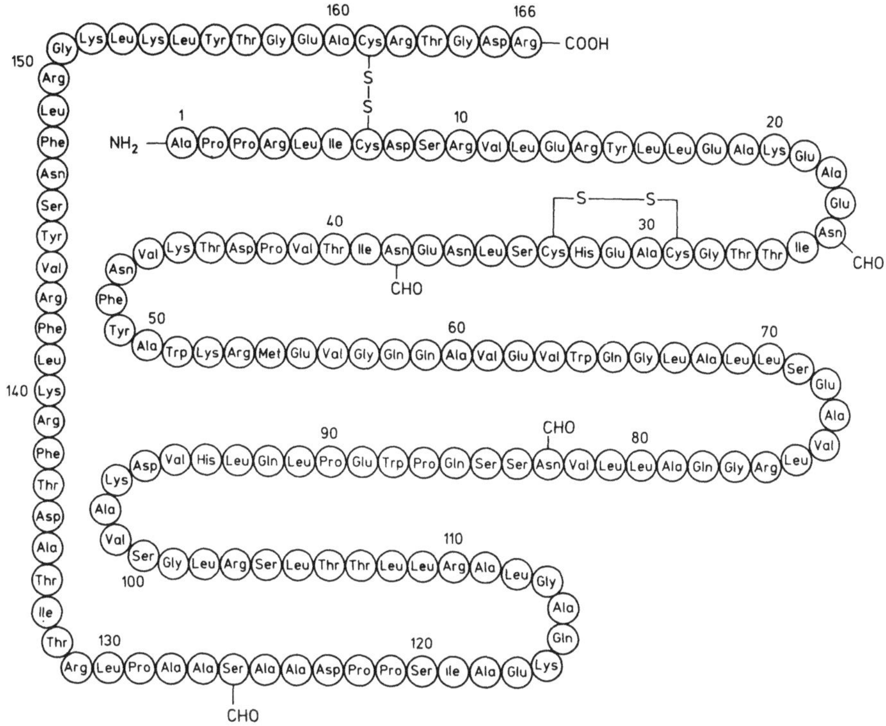

Fig. 1. The primary amino acid sequence of human erythropoietin. The sequence is folded arbitrarily for illustration. Two disulphide bonds link Cys 7 with Cys 161 and Cys 29 with Cys 33. The three N-linked glycosylation sites occur at aspartyl residues 24, 38 and 83. One O-linked glycosylation site is present at Ser 126

terminal regions are relatively highly charged. Glycyl and prolyl residues are known to inhibit strongly the formation of α-helix and β-sheet structures, and because regions 4–27 and 130–150 are deficient in these amino acids, they may contain α-helical structures [15].

Human Epo contains four cysteine residues [20]. Lai et al. [15] havc deduced from Edman degradation studies of tryptic and V8 protease fragments that human Epo contains two disulphide bonds, one between Cys 7 and Cys 161 and the other between Cys 29 and Cys 33, as shown in Fig. 1. The latter bond completes the formation of a small flat loop of five residues. In mouse Epo residue 33 is a proline instead of a cysteine [21] but the secondary structure analysis by the method of Chou and Fasman [22] indicates the same type of flat loop, suggesting that this area is probably important for biological function [23].

Human Epo contains four glycosylation sites (see Fig. 1). Three of these are N-glycosylation sites at positions 24, 38 and 83, dictated by the consenus glycosylation sequence, Asn-X-Ser/Thr [24]. Dordal et al. [25], using the enzyme endoglycosidase F which removes asparagine-linked sugars, demonstrated that a major proportion of the carbohydrate of Epo is asparagine – or N-linked. Egrie et al. [26] extended this work and, using a combination of N- and O-glycanases, demonstrated that Epo contained an O-linked as well as three N-linked oligosaccharide chains. The fourth carbohydrate chain is O-linked to the seryl residue 126, based on the detection of galactosamine, the N-acetylated ester of which is the linking sugar to hydroxyamino acids [15, 27].

Secondary Protein Structure

Investigation of the secondary structure of Epo by circular dichroism (CD) indicated that it has an α-helical content of 50% and that the remainder of the molecule has a mainly random configuration with no evidence for β-sheet structure [15]. Partial proteolysis of Epo, containing ^{3}H-labelled sialic acid incorporated in the oligosaccharide chains, resulted in the formation of two trypsin-resistant domains each with an apparent Nr of approximately 16000 and a small trypsin-sensitive region [20]. None of the tryptic fragments had biological activity [20].

Carbohydrate Structure

Purified U-Epo consists of two froms (α and β) which have similar specific activities in vivo [12] although their overall carbohydrate content differs [25]. Desialation, which involves the removal of neuramininic acid from Epo, results in increased activity in vitro [28]. Similarly, enzymatic deglycosylation of Epo produces a mixture of aggregated forms and a monomer. The aggregated forms have no biological activity but the monomer has enhanced biological activity in vitro [23]. After desialation or deglycosylation activity in vivo is completely lost [29]. The hydrophilic oligosaccharide structures may maintain the conformation of the hydrophobic polypeptide structure but may not be directly involved in the interaction with cellular receptors for Epo [23].

The oligosaccharide structure also affects the turnover rate and antigenicity of Epo [25, 28 31] in addition to its effect on bioactivity. In view of the proposed therapeutic use of rHu Epo, it was important to elucidate the oligosaccharide structure for comparison with the native human form.

The carbohydrate compositions of human U-Epo and rHu Epo derived from several cell types [25, 32, 33] are shown in Table 1. A comparison of the molar carbohydrate composition of U-Epo reported by the three groups of workers shows good agreement. U-Epo and recombinant Epo isolated from CHO cells are strikingly similar in sugar content [32]. The N-acetylneuraminic acid composition of the recombinant Epos shows a 3.7-fold variation ranging from 5.0 moles/mole in r Epo τ to 18.7 moles/mole in r Epo-B. The r Epo-τ variant exhibited only 25% of the biological activity in vivo shown by the more sialated Epos [33].

The oligosaccharide chains in U-Epo and rHu Epo produced by CHO cells are similar [32, 34] except for the sialyl-galactosyl linkage [34]. Recombinant Hu Epo

Table 1. Molar carbohydrate composition of various erythropoietins

Sugar	Sugar content (moles/mole of Epo)						
	(i) U-Epo α	(ii) U-Epo β	(iii) U-Epo	(iv) r Epo	(v) U-Epo	(vi) r Epo B	(vii) r Epo τ
Fucose	4 ± 0.8	4 ± 0.1	2.9	3.2	2.6	3.3	3.2
Galactose	11 ± 1.4	11 ± 0.1	12.9	14.1	13.3	15.7	20.6
Mannose	9 ± 1.2	8 ± 1.0	9.2	8.9	8.1	10.1	11.4
N-Acetylglucosamine	12 ± 0.2	9 ± 0.6	17.2	19.4	22.1	28.9	26.8
N-Acetylneuraminic acid	16 ± 2.2	12 ± 1.0	10.4	10.5	10.7	18.7	5.0

Data in columns (i) and (ii) from Dordal et al. [25]; columns (iii) and (iv) recalculated from Sasaki et al. [32] and columns (v), (vi) and (vii) from Goto et al. [33]

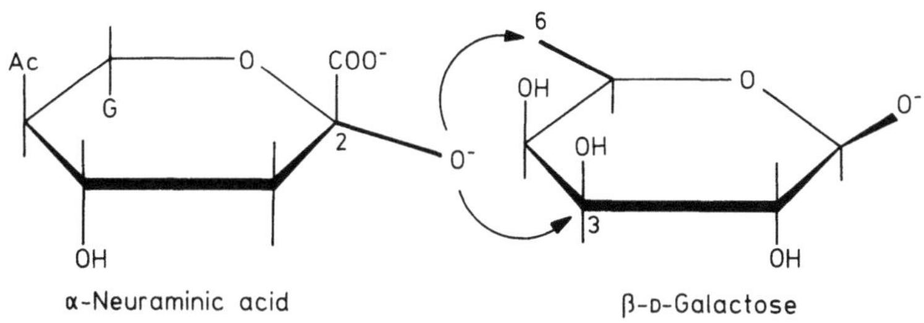

Fig. 2. Configuration of N-acetylneuraminic acid-galactose bonds in erythropoietin. Recombinant human Epo and U-Epo both contain the N-acetylneuraminic acid 2→3 galactose linkage. In addition U-Epo contains the N-acetylneuraminic acid 2→6 galactose linkage. *Ac*, acetamido group; *G*, glycerol group

and U-Epo both contain an N-acetylneuraminic acid 2→3 galactose linkage. The U-Epo contains in addition an N-acetylneuraminic acid 2→6 galactose linkage. Both types of linkage are illustrated in Fig. 2. One O-linked oligosaccharide chain is present in both U-Epo and in rHu Epo [32].

A large proportion of the carbohydrate structure of rHu Epo isolated from CHO cells is composed of triantennary and tetraantennary saccharide [32]. For the N-linked oligosaccharide, only 1.4% of the total saccharide was in biantennary structures, compared to 13.5% in triantennary and 85.1% in tetra-antennary structures. Rat liver cells take up the desialated form of glycoproteins which contain tri- and tetra-antennary oligosaccharides [35], and this is consistent with the observation that desialated Epo is taken up by liver cells through a galactose-binding protein [28]. Sasaki et al. [32] have pointed out that sialylation of administered Epo by 2→6 sialyltransferase may extend its half-life in the circulation.

Assays of Erythropoietin

Introduction

The purification of human U-Epo by Miyake et al. in 1977 marked a turning point in the assay of Epo because it made possible the development of reliable radioimmunoassays for Epo [36, 37]. Until rHu Epo became available the supply of pure Epo was severely limited and therefore in vivo and in vitro assays were widely used.

In Vivo Assays

Early assays for Epo relied upon animals in which erythropoiesis had been experimentally suppressed, for example fasted rats [38] and mice made polycythaemic either by transfusion [39] or by exposure to hypoxia followed by return to normal oxygen tension [40]. These animals were thus made more sensitive to erythropoietic stimuli. Injection of such animals with Epo followed by ^{59}Fe causes a dose-dependent incorporation of the isotope into the circulating red blood cells. The minimum detectable dose for the fasted rat assay is 1 U of Epo, and for the polycythaemic and ex-hypoxic mouse assays it is approximately 50 mU. In vivo assays are therefore not sensitive enough to measure normal circulating plasma Epo. In addition they are imprecise, time-consuming and labour-intensive.

In Vitro Assays

Several in vitro assays have been developed using cells from a variety of sources in primary explant culture. Such assays, capable of detecting 1 to 5 mU of Epo and therefore considerably more sensitive than in vivo assays, have been developed with rat bone marrow cells using ^{59}Fe incorporation into haem [41] and fetal mouse liver cells using labelled thymidine incorporation into DNA [42]. In a variant of the latter type, ^{3}H-uridine incorporation was used to monitor stimulation of RNA synthesis by Epo in 12-day-old fetal mouse liver proerythroblasts [43].

An assay procedure using spleen cells from mice which had previously been made anaemic by the administration of phenylhydrazine has been described by Krystal [44]. Low concentrations of Epo (approximately 3 mU/ml) cause a significant increase in DNA synthesis which is readily monitored by incorporation of labelled thymidine into the DNA of proliferating cells. An important advantage of the mouse spleen cell assay (MSCA) is that several hundred assays can be performed using spleen cells from one animal.

In vitro assays are affected by non-specific factors present in serum. For example, estimates of serum Epo using bioassays are influenced by other growth factors and hormones present in the serum matrix [45]. The MSCA is affected by the percentage saturation of the transferrin with iron [46]. Human serum can be toxic to cells in vitro due to the presence of IgM-related heteroantibodies. This toxicity can be removed by heat treatment at 56 °C for 30 min [47] but this process destroys some of the Epo.

Radioimmunoassays

Introduction

Radioimmunoassays (RIAs) are usually more specific, sensitive, precise and convenient than bioassays and are now generally preferred for the measurement of serum Epo. The development of an RIA procedure requires: (1) the availability of pure Epo for radiolabelling; (2) a specific antibody to Epo; and (3) a technique for the separation of hormone which has bound to the antibody from hormone which has not bound to the antibody.

Radiolabelling Of Epo Tracer For RIA

The availability of purified U-Epo and more recently of rHu Epo has made feasible the widespread use of RIAs. Radioactive iodine is incorporated into the tyrosyl residues of Epo using a variety of reagents which release iodine from ^{125}I-iodide. These include the chloramine T reagent developed by Hunter and Greenwood [48], the two-phase chloramine T procedure of Tejedor and Ballestra [49] and the water-insoluble reagent 1,3,4,6-tetrachloro-3a,6a-diphenylglycouril (Iodo-gen, Pierce Chemical Company) used in the method of Fraker and Speck [50]. Specific activities of 50–455μCi/μg Epo have been obtained using chloramine T [51, 52] and Iodo-gen [36, 53 – 55]. This range corresponds to 0.7–6.5 nCi/mU and to an incorporation of 0.6–8 atoms of ^{125}I per molecule of Epo. A procedure using lactoperoxidase to iodinate Epo [5] produced material with specific activity of 55–128 μCi/μg. ^{125}I-labelled Epo with a specific activity of approximately 10 μCi/μg is commercially available from Amersham International Ltd.

Antibodies Required For RIA

Polyclonal antibodies from rabbits are generally employed for RIA and are often raised to relatively crude Epo preparations. The use of rHu Epo for antibody production has also been reported [56]. Antisera should have a high titre and exhibit strong affinity for the antigen. Ideally they should also have equal affinity for both the labelled and unlabelled form of the antigen to give satisfactory displacement kinetics. However, this ideal is seldom achieved in practice, and disequilibrium systems, where the addition of labelled Epo has been delayed for periods ranging from 2 to 72 h, have been described [5, 55–57]. Separation of antibody-bound hormone from non-bound hormone is usually achieved with goat anti-rabbit gamma globulin with added rabbit serum as carrier.

Estimation of Erythropoietin in Serum

Cotes [58] has compared 20 separately published estimates of serum Epo concentrations and found that the ranges (or calculated 95% confidence intervals of these estimates) spanned concentrations from 2.5 to 4000 mU/ml (1 to 1000 pmol/l). These estimates were probably based on methods with different specificities or in some cases on standards with values which had been wrongly assigned.

Although the polycythaemic mouse bioassay is not sensitive enough for the estimation of normal plasma Epo concentrations, Erslev and his colleagues [59] used the assay to measure preconcentrated plasma Epo extracts. With this technique they found a mean normal plasma Epo concentration of 7.8 mU/ml compared with a value of less than 5 mU/ml for a group of patients with polycythaemia vera. Dunn and Lange [60], in a review of in vitro bioassays, suggest a value of 40 mU/ml for normal serum using the in vitro fetal mouse liver cell assay, in close agreement with de Klerk et al. [61], who obtained a mean of 38 mU/ml for normal sera. Lappin et al. [57], using the mouse spleen cell assay, established a normal range of 43 ± 15 mU/ml (mean ± 1SD). The same samples, when measured by RIA, resulted in a normal range of 17 ± 6 mU/ml. This range for RIA is in reasonable agreement with the results of Koeffler and Goldwasser [3] and Garcia et al. [4].

Garcia et al. [4], using an RIA similar to that used by Koeffler and Goldwasser [3], found a slightly higher mean Epo level in normal females (18.8 mU/ml) than normal males (17.2 mU/ml). Mean plasma Epo concentrations in male and female patients with polycythaemia vera were 9.2 and 8.7 mU/ml respectively, significantly lower than normal. Male and female patients with secondary polycythaemia had significantly increased mean serum Epo concentrations of 153.7 and 75.7 mU/ml respectively. Koeffler and Goldwasser [3] found that 92% of patients with polycythaemia vera had concentrations less than 30 mU/ml, whereas 94% of patients with secondary polycythaemia had concentrations greater than 30 mU/ml. This criterion taken alone gave them a 93% correct classification of the polycythaemic conditions, thereby demonstrating the usefulness of the RIA in distinguishing, in most cases, between polycythaemia vera and secondary polycythaemia. Cotes and her colleagues [62] have pointed out that a measurement of the serum Epo in a single sample may not always discriminate between these two conditions, because the elevated serum Epo may occur intermittently.

In anaemic patients, whose condition is not complicated by renal or chronic disease, serum Epo levels are often high, and values of the order of 1000 to 10000 mU/ml have been reported in aplastic anaemia [55, 59].

In the anaemia of chronic renal failure (CRF), serum Epo levels ascertained by RIA are generally similar to or slightly higher than those in normal non-anaemic controls [63, 64]. When measured by RIA the levels are usually 75–100% higher than in non-anaemic subjects and higher than those found by bioassay [64–66]. However, in CRF, serum Epo levels are generally lower than those in other patients with comparable haemoglobin concentrations. Urabe et al. [55] found significantly lower levels of serum Epo in patients with CRF (mean ± SD 26.6 ± 3.8 mU/ml) than in those with anaemia of equal severity due to iron deficiency (80.3 ± 17.3 mU/ml).

Discrepancies in serum Epo levels determined by RIA and the plethoric mouse assay suggested that immunoreactive Epo with little or no biological activity may be present in the serum of CRF patients [36]. Recent studies have demonstrated that Epo in the sera of normal and uraemic subjects is heterogeneous and consists of three components with different immunoreactivities [67]. These components have molecular weights lower than, equal to and higher than native Epo as determined by fractionation on a gel permeation column. These findings warrant further study, since only the component with a molecular weight similar to native Epo was found to have biological activity.

References

1. Goldwasser E (1975) Erythropoietin and the differentiation of red blood cells. Fed Proc 34: 2285–2292
2. Graber SE, Krantz SB (1978) Erythropoietin and the control of red cell production. Annu Rev Med 29: 51–66
3. Koeffler HP, Goldwasser E (1981) Erythropoietin radioimmunoassay in evaluating patients with polycythemia. Ann Intern Med 94: 44–47
4. Garcia JF, Ebbe SN, Hollander L, Cutting HO, Miller ME, Cronkite EP (1982) Radioimmunoassay of erythropoietin: circulating levels in normal and polycythemic human beings. J Lab Clin Med 99: 624–635
5. Cotes PM (1982) Immunoreactive erythropoietin in serum. 1. Evidence for the validity of the assay method and the physiological relevance of estimates. Br J Haematol 50: 427–438
6. Davis JM, Arakawa T, Strickland TW, Yphantis DA (1987) Characterization of recombinant human erythropoietin produced in Chinese hamster ovary cells. Biochemistry 26: 2633–2638
7. Mok M, Spivak JL (1982) Protease activity in human urine erythropoietin preparations. Exp Hematol 10: 300–306
8. Lowy PH (1970) Preparation and chemistry of erythropoietin. In: Gordon AS (ed) Regulation of hematopoiesis. Appleton-Century-Crofts, East Norwalk, pp 395–412
9. Espada J, Brandan NC, Dorado M (1973) Effect of chemical and enzymatic agents on the biological activity of erythropoietin. Acta Physiol Latinoam 23: 193–201
10. Lee-Huang S (1980) A new preparative method for isolation of human erythropoietin with hydrophobic interaction chromatography. Blood 56: 620–624
11. Wang FF, Kung CK-H, Goldwasser E (1985) Some chemical properties of human erythropoietin. Endocrinology 116: 2286–2292
12. Miyake T, Kung CK-H, Goldwasser E (1977) Purification of human erythropoietin. J Biol Chem 252: 5558–5564
13. Lin F-K, Suggs S, Lin C-H, Browne JK, Smalling R, Egrie JC, Chen KK, Fox GM, Martin F, Stabinsky Z, Badrawi SM, Lai P-H, Goldwasser E (1985) Cloning and expression of the human erythropoietin gene. Proc Natl Acad Sci USA 82: 7580–7584

14. Jacobs K, Shoemaker C, Rudersdorf R, Neill SD, Kaufmann RJ, Mufson A, Seehra J, Jones SS, Hewick R, Fritsch EF, Kawakita M, Shimizu T, Miyake T (1985) Isolation and characterization of genomic and cDNA clones of human erythropoietin. Nature 313: 806–810
15. Lai P-H, Everett R, Wang F-F, Arakawa T, Goldwasser E (1986) Structural characterization of human erythropoietin. J Biol Chem 261: 3116–3121
16. Fyhrquist F, Rosenlöf K, Grönhagen-Riska C, Hortling L, Tikkanen I (1984) Is renin substrate an erythropoietin precursor? Nature 308: 649–652
17. Powell JS, Berker KL, Lebo RV, Adamson JW (1986) Human erythropoietin gene: high level expression in stably transfected mammalian cells and chromosome localization. Proc Natl Acad Sci USA 83: 6465–6469
18. Watkins PC, Eddy R, Hoffman N, Stranislovitis P, Beck AK, Galli J, Vellucci V, Gusella JF, Shows TB (1986) Regional assignment of the erythropoietin gene to human chromosome region 7pter – q22. Cytogenet Cell Genet 42: 214–218
19. Recny MA, Scoble HA, Kim Y (1987) Structural characterization of natural human urinary and recombinant DNA – derived erythropoietin. J Biol Chem 262: 17156–17163
20. Wang FF, Kung CK-H, Goldwasser E (1985) Some chemical properties of human erythropoietin. Endocrinology 116: 2286–2292
21. McDonald JD, Lin F-K, Goldwasser E (1986) Cloning, sequencing and evolutionary analysis of the mouse erythropoietin gene. Mol Cell Biol 6: 842–848
22. Chou PY, Fasman GD (1978) Empirical predictions of protein conformation. Annu Rev Biochem 47: 251–276
23. Goldwasser E, McDonald J, Beru N (1987) The molecular biology of erythropoietin and the expression of its gene. In: Rich IN (ed) Molecular and cellular aspects of erythropoietin and erythropoiesis. Springer, Berlin Heidelberg New York pp 11–21 (NATO ASI series, vol H8)
24. Neuberger A, Gottschalk A, Marshall RD, Spiro RG (1972) Carbohydrate-peptide linkages in glycoproteins and methods for their elucidation. In: Gottschalk A (ed) The glycoproteins: their composition, structure and function. Elsevier/North Holland, Amsterdam, pp 450–490
25. Dordal MS, Wang FF, Goldwasser E (1985) The role of carbohydrate in erythropoietin action. Endocrinology 116: 2293–2299
26. Egrie JC, Strickland TW, Lane J, Aoki K, Cohen AM, Smalling R, Trail G, Lin FK, Browne JK, Hinds DK (1986) Characterization and biological effects of recombinant human erythropoietin. Immunobiol ogy 172: 213–224
27. Takeuchi M, Takasaki S, Inoue N, Kobata A (1988) Sensitive method for carbohydrate composition analysis of glycoproteins by high-performance liquid chromatography. J Chromatogr 400: 207–213
28. Goldwasser E, Kung CK-H, Eliason JF (1974) On the mechanism of erythropoietin-induced differentiation. 13. The role of sialic acid in erythropoietin action. J Biol Chem 249: 4202–4206
29. Lowy PH, Keighley G, Borsook H (1960) Inactivation of erythropoietin by neuraminidase and by mild substitution reactions. Nature 185: 102–103
30. Briggs DW, Fisher JW, George WJ (1974) Hepatic clearance of intact and desialylated erythropoietin. Am J Physiol 227: 1385–1388
31. Schooley JC (1985) Neuraminidase increases DNA synthesis of spleen cells induced by native and asialylated erythropoietin. Exp Hematol 13: 994–998
32. Sasaki H, Bothner B, Dell A, Fukuda M (1987) Carbohydrate structure of erythropoietin expressed in Chinese hamster ovary cells by a human erythropoietin cDNA. J Biol Chem 262: 12059–12076
33. Goto M, Akai K, Murakami A, Hashimoto C, Tsuda E, Ueda M, Kawanishi G, Takahashi N, Ishimoto A, Chiba H, Sasaki R (1988) Production of recombinant human erythropoietin in mammalian cells: host cell dependency of the biological activity of the cloned glycoprotein. Biotechnology 6: 67–71
34. Takeuchi M, Takasaki S, Miyazaki H, Kato T, Hoshi S, Kochibe N, Kobata A (1988) Comparative study of the asparagine – linked sugar chains of human erythropoietins purified

from urine and the culture medium of recombinant Chinese hamster ovary cells. J Biol Chem 263: 3657–3663
35. Morell AG, Irvine RA, Sternlieb I, Scheinberg IH, Ashwell G (1968) Physical and chemical studies on ceruloplasmin in vivo. J Biol Chem 243: 155–159
36. Sherwood JB, Goldwasser E (1979) A radioimmunoassay for erythropoietin. Blood 54: 885–893
37. Garcia JF, Sherwood JB, Goldwasser E (1979) Radioimmunoassay of erythropoietin. Blood Cells 5: 405–419
38. Fried W, Plzak LF, Jacobson LO, Goldwasser E (1957) Studies on erythropoiesis. III. Factors controlling erythropoietin production. Proc Soc Exp Biol Med 94: 237–241
39. Jacobson LO, Goldwasser E, Plzak LF, Fried W (1957) Studies on erythropoiesis. IV. Reticulocyte response of hypophysectomized and polycythemic rodents to erythropoietin. Proc Soc Exp Biol Med 94: 243–249
40. Cotes PM, Bangham DR (1961) Bioassay of erythropoietin in mice made polycythaemic by exposure to air at reduced pressure. Nature 191: 1065–1067
41. Goldwasser E, Eliason JF, Sikkema D (1975) An assay for erythropoietin in vitro at the milliunit level. Endocrinology 97: 315–323
42. Dunn CDR, Jarvis JH, Greenman JM (1975) A quantitative bioassay for erythropoietin using mouse fetal liver cells. Exp Hematol 3: 65–78
43. Bessler H, Notti I, Djaldetti M (1980) Quantitative determination of human plasma erythropoietin using embryonic mouse liver erythroblasts. Acta Haematol 63: 204–210
44. Krystal G (1983) A simple microassay for erythropoietin based on ^{3}H-thymidine incorporation into spleen cells from phenylhydrazine – treated mice. Exp Hematol 11: 649–660
45. Sherwood JB (1984) The chemistry and physiology of erythropoietin. Academic, New York pp 161–211, Vitamins and hormones, vol 41
46. Lappin TRJ, Elder GE, McKibbin SH, McNamee PT, McGeown MG, Bridges JM (1985) The effect of transferrin saturation on the estimation of erythropoietin by the mouse spleen cell microassay. Exp Hematol 13: 1007–1013
47. Goldwasser E (1973) Erythropoietin. Methods in investigative and diagnostic endocrinology, p III, nonpituitary hormones. Elsevier, Amsterdam, p 1097
48. Hunter WM, Greenwod FC (1962) Preparation of iodine – ^{131}I-labelled human growth hormone of high specific activity. Nature 194: 495–496
49. Tejedor G, Ballestra JPG (1982) Iodination of biological samples without loss of functional activity. Anal Biochem 127: 143–149
50. Fraker PJ, Speck Jr JC (1978) Protein and cell membrane iodinations with a sparingly soluble chloroamide, 1,3,4,6-tetrachloro-3a,6a-diphenylglycoluril. Biochem Biophys Res Commun 80: 849–857
51. Rege AB, Brookins J, Fisher JW (1982) A radioimmunoassay for erythropoietin: serum levels in normal human subjects and patients with hemopoietic disorders. J Lab Clin Med 100: 829–843
52. Garcia JF, Clemons GK (1983) The radioimmunoassay of erythropoietin. In: Lawrence JH, Winchell S (eds) Recent advances in nuclear medicine, vol 6. Grune and Stratton, New York, pp 19–40.
53. Sawyer ST, Krantz SB, Goldwasser E (1987) Binding and Receptor – mediated endocytosis of erythropoietin in Friend Virus – infected erythroid cells. J Biol Chem 262: 5554–5562
54. Mizoguchi H, Ohta K, Suzuki T, Murakami A, Ueda M, Sasaki R, Chiba H (1987) Basic conditions for radioimmunoassay of erythropoietin, and plasma levels of erythropoietin in normal subjects and anaemic patients. Acta Haematol Jpn 50: 15–24
55. Urabe A, Saito T, Fukamachi H, Kubota M, Takaku F (1987) Serum erythropoietin titers in the anemia of chronic renal failure and other hematological states. Int J Cell Cloning 5: 202–208
56. Egrie JC, Lane J (1987) Development of a radioimmunoassay for erythropoietin using recombinant erythropietin – derived reagents. In: Rich IN (ed) Molecular and cellular aspects of erythropoietin and erythropoiesis. Springer, Berlin Heidelberg New York pp 395–407 (NATO ASI series, vol H8)

57. Lappin TRJ, Elder GE, Taylor T, McMullin MF, Bridges JM (1988) Comparison of the mouse spleen cell assay and a radioimmunoassay for the measurement of serum erythropoietin. Br J Haematol 70: 117–120
58. Cotes PM (1987) The estimation of erythropoietin (Epo): principles, problems and progress. In: Rich IN (ed) Molecular and cellular aspects of erythropoietin and erythropoiesis. Springer, Berlin Heidelberg New York pp 377–387 (NATO ASI series, vol H8)
59. Erslev AJ, Wilson J, Caro J (1987) Erythropoietin titers in anemic nonuremic patients. J Lab Clin Med 109: 429–433
60. Dunn CDR, Lange RD (1980) Erythropoietin titers in normal human serum. An appraisal of assay techniques. Exp Hematol 8: 231–235
61. de Klerk G, Vet RJ, Rosengarten PC, Goudsmit R (1980) Comparison of the hemagglutination inhibition assay kit for erythropoietin (ESF) with the fetal mouse liver cell bioassy in vitro. Blood 55: 955–959
62. Cotes PM, Doré CJ, Liu Yin JA, Lewis SM, Messinezy M, Pearson TC, Reid C (1986) Determination of serum immunoreactive erythropoietin in the investigation of erythrocytosis. N Engl J Med 315: 283–287
63. Caro J, Brown S, Miller O, Murray T, Erslev AJ (1979) Erythropoietin levels in uremic nephric and anephric patients. J Lab Clin Med 93: 449–458
64. Zaroulis CG, Hoffman BJ, Kourides IA (1981) Serum concentrations of erythropoietin measured by radioimmunoassay in hematologic disorders and chronic renal failure. Am J Hematol 11: 85–92
65. Fisher JW, Lertora JL, Lindholm DD, Tornyos K, Moriyama Y (1973) Erythropoietin production and inhibitors in serum in the anemia of uremia. Proc Clin Dialysis Transplant Forum 3: 22–23
66. McGonigle RJS, Husserl F, Wallin JD, Fisher JW (1984) Hemodialysis and continuous ambulatory peritoneal dialysis effects on erythropoiesis in renal failure. Kidney Int 25: 430–436
67. Sherwood JB, Carmichael LD, Goldwasser E (1988) The heterogeneity of circulating human serum erythropoietin. Endocrinology 122: 1472–1477

Erythropoietin Production Under Steady-State Conditions: Detection and Localization Using In Situ Hybridization*

I. N. RICH

Introduction

The original observation by Jacobson et al. in 1957 [1] that the kidney can produce erythropoietin under hypoxic conditions, has been recently substantiated by molecular biology techniques [2–8]. Northern transfer analysis with DNA [2–6, 8] and RNA [7] probes, and in situ hybridization [7–9] were employed for this purpose. From these investigations however, a more important, but overlooked, observation is now also clear; little or no erythropoietin production occurs in the kidney under normal, steady-state conditions [2–9].

The function of the kidney in erythropoietin production appears, therefore, to occur under stress or pathophysiological conditions. Since the day-to-day production of erythropoietin is the rule rather than the exception, several important aspects of the physiology of erythropoietin production and erythropoiesis need clarification. Some of the open questions pertaining to erythropoietin production are listed in Table 1 and briefly reviewed and discussed in this presentation.

Erythropoietin production is dependent on the prevailing partial oxygen tension delivered by the erythrocytes. The mechanism for measuring partial oxygen tension by the biological sensor is unknown. Similarly, there is no information on how the signal is transferred into an increase or decrease in erythropoietin production. Under normal conditions, the pO_2 at the cellular location site of erythropoietin production, is lower than that present in the venous system (approx. 45 mmHg). This is due to the presence of oxygen gradients resulting in pO_2 values in the range of 15–45 mmHg or lower. Assuming this to be the situation under normal conditions, what happens under hypoxic or other stress conditions where the initial pO_2 is much lower? Is the pO_2 reaching the erythropoietin oxygen sensor decreased to such an extent that such extreme conditions cannot be properly transferred into a response? If not, is this reason for erythropoietin production being transferred to other organs? There is no information to shed any light on these possible processes. Yet signals must be present which regulate the site and production of

* This work was supported by the German Red Cross and the Deutsche Forschungsgemeinschaft.

Table 1. Ten questions on erythropoietin production

1. What is the erythropoietin oxygen sensor?
2. Are oxygen sensing and erythropoietin production performed in the same cell?
3. What is the range of pO_2 that the oxygen sensor can withstand, or is it open ended?
4. How is the signal for pO_2 determined on the cell surface – if it is in fact determined there?
5. What ist the mechanism of cellular internalization of a cellular pO_2 signal?
6. What are the intracellular mechanisms whereby the signal is transferred into the control of erythropoietin production? For example, does this occur at the genetic, translation, glycosylation or packaging stage of erythropoietin production?
7. Where is erythropoietin produced during ontogeny?
8. Where is erythropoietin produced under normal steady-state conditions?
9. Under stress or pathophysiological conditions, are all hemopoietic organs involved in erythropoietin production, or is the latter dependent on the severity of the condition?
10. What ist the mechanism by which erythropoietin production is transferred to other organs during stress or pathophysiological conditions?

erythropoietin under normal conditions. These may be defective, masked or inhibited, or even absent under pathophysiological conditions.

Considering our meager knowledge of the erythropoietin oxygen sensor, it may take many years before we can even begin to understand how this phenomenon occurs. In other areas, however, there is no doubt that molecular biology has provided us with an extremely powerful and sophisticated tool with which to answer some of the questions raised in Table 1. The questions involving cellular localization of erythropoietin gene expression under normal steady-state conditions are best investigated using in situ hybridization.

In Situ Hybridization

Nearly all the information accrued so far on erythropoietin gene expression has involved Northern transfer analysis. This very sensitive technique (1 pg of specific RNA) allows quantitation, analysis of specificity of the probe and determination of the presence of specific RNA. However, unless one is working with homogeneous cell lines, Northern transfer does not provide any information concerning the cell type and location of the cell or cells involved in RNA synthesis in organs, tissues or heterogeneous cell suspensions.

If using radioactive probes, in situ hybridization can also be quantitated to a certain extent. However, the principal advantage of this technique is the morphological identification and location of cells expressing a specific message. Coupled with the possibility of performing multiple labelling techniques on the same preparation, information is obtained which would not be available using Northern transfer.

For many years in situ hybridization has been based on the autoradiographic signal detection system using DNA or RNA probes labelled with ^{3}H, ^{35}S, ^{32}P, ^{125}I. Many investigators assume that radiolabels provide the greatest sensitivity. This is not necessarily the case. There are also many obvious disadvantages to using radioactivity.

There is now an increasing trend toward the use of nonradioactive probes for both Northern transfer and in situ hybridization. Target sequences detected with biotinylated probes for instance, have similar sensitivity to radiolabelled probes (1–5 pg). Compared to radioactive probes, non-radioactive probes are easier to use (no need for special laboratories and precautions, not to mention taking the half-life of the radiolabel into account), can be produced in bulk and allow rapid results.

At least three different types of non-radioactive labels for in situ hybridization studies exist: (a) indirect or direct fluorescence-labelled probes [10–13], (b) mercurate-labelled probes, which are also observed by fluorescence [14–16] and (c) biotinylated probes [17–26] which can be detected by immunohistochemical means in which the final signal is either enzymatic (e.g. peroxidase, alkaline phosphatase) or electron dense (e.g. colloidal gold).

Localization of specific gene expression on a per cell basis is the primary objective of in situ hybridization. To this end, a balance must be obtained between sensitivity of the signal detecting gene expression and cellular morphology. There are many protocols available for the in situ hybridization technique. These involve either aqueous or non-aqueous (using formamide) conditions, low (37 °C) or high (42 °C) hybridization temperature and low, moderate or high stringency conditions. In addition, a denaturation and/or dehydration step is usually included. We have found that denaturation and dehydration are particularly harmful and do not allow morphological identification of the cells involved in gene expression. For this reason, we omit these steps completely. However, in general, the method one employs is dependent on the type of cells and the type of probe being used. This means that the final protocol is usually obtained by trial and error.

An important aspect of in situ hybridization using non-radioactive-labelled probes is the almost complete absence of background. Radioactive-labelled probes usually produce a good deal of background due to inherent radioactive emission distances. This is not usually the case with non-radioactive probes, although the presence of background also depends on the conditions used before and after hybridization. To reduce background, all slides are nitric acid washed and pyrolyzed through a flame. The preparations are acetylated [27] and treated with glycine. After hybridization, the preparations are washed with Tween 80 to reduce adhesion of the signal detection system to the glass. All these conditions have been described in detail elsewhere and are specific for detection of erythropoietin gene expression in vitro and in vivo, using a biotin-labelled erythropoietin DNA probe [9, 28].

Steady-State Production of Erythropoietin

For a continuous production rate of 10^{12}–10^{13} erythrocytes per day, a continuous stimulus must be present. If this signal was emanating from the kidney, erythropoietin gene expression should be detectable. The inability to detect erythropoietin gene expression in the kidney under normal conditions implies that the hormone must be produced elsewhere.

Considerable information is available showing that the macrophage plays an important role in erythropoiesis. This information is summarized in Table 2. Our interest in the macrophage is not, however, limited to its possible role in erythropoiesis, but includes its role as a regulator cell for hemopoiesis in general [35–37]. Because erythropoietin and erythropoiesis are extremely well characterized, we have concentrated our studies on erythropoietin production.

We have argued that under normal steady-state conditions, the macrophage could have the functional ability to produce and secrete erythropoietin at the sites of erythropoiesis [36–39]. This hypothesis was tested first using an almost pure population of macrophages derived by culturing unseparated and unstimulated normal mouse bone marrow cells on hydrophobic Teflon foils for 14 days. These cells were then subjected to in situ hybridization using a 1.2–kb erythropoietin DNA probe. In the initial experiments, the DNA was labelled using ^{35}S-dUTP [28]. Not only was it possible to detect erythropoietin gene expression in these cultured cells, but by labelling the cells using a monoclonal antibody directed against the mouse, macrophage-specific F4/80 antigen, it was possible to show that the macrophage, and not a contaminating cell population, was expressing the gene.

Experiments performed in parallel using the radioactive in situ hybridization technique employed the biotin-labelled erythropoietin DNA. The signal was determined using a streptavidin-biotin-peroxidase complex. Although an apparent specific hybridization was obtained (not all the cells were labelled), this enzymatic signal proved difficult to use due to endogenous peroxidase activity and the low

Table 2. Findings showing the important role of the macrophage in erythropoiesis

1. The macrophage is one of the first, if not the first morphologically identifiable hemopoietic cell to colonize the fetal liver [29].
2. The macrophage is the source of fetal liver erythropoietin [30].
3. In fetal liver, macrophages are present as "central cells" or "nurse cells" in erythroid blood islands.
4. The erythropoietin-producing function of the fetal liver is carried over to the adult liver.
5. The Kupffer cell can release erythropoietin [31].
6. Erythropoietin can be released from fetal liver, adult liver, kidney, bone marrow and spleen by incubation of the suspension with the macrophage-specific, cytotoxic agent, crystalline silica [32].
7. Release of erythropoietin from bone marrow and spleen cells by crystalline silica is dependent on the in vivo oxygen tension [32].
8. "Erythroid blood islands" can be isolated and identified from the adult bone marrow [33, 34].

colour development [28]. Similar in situ hybridization experiments using biotinylated erythropoietin DNA and a streptavidin-alkaline phosphatase signal detection system improved the sensitivity somewhat, but again colour development of the enzymatic reaction proved to be a problem.

We turned next to gold as a signal for non-radioactive in situ hybridization. For several reasons, this has turned out to be the method of choice. Gold can be viewed as a signal both under normal and electron microscopy. Under bright-field microscopy, the signal appears as brown particle aggregates. Gold particles are obtained in various defined sizes as well as being conjugated to other carrier or binding molecules. Finally, gold can reflect the light allowing visualization under the reflection-contrast microscope. The latter was originally developed to view the adherence of cells on different surfaces [40, 41].

Recent studies have therefore concentrated on using biotinylated erythropoietin DNA coupled with streptavidin-gold signal detection and visualization under the reflection-contrast microscope. The results using cultured macrophages confirmed the original studies using radiolabelled erythropoietin DNA [28]. In fact, the non-radioactive in situ hybridization studies have shown that of the 98% population of macrophages present after 14 days, about 34% express both the erythropoietin gene and the F4/80 antigen, indicating that a subpopulation of macrophages is responsible for this function [9, 39]. The specificity of the signal has been determined by RNA dot-blot analysis using both total and poly(A)$^+$ RNA from kidney from severely anemic mice and 14-day-cultured macrophages [39]. Further specificity of the in situ hybridization technique is shown using a biotin-labelled actin DNA probe [39].

However, probably the most important observation from these non-radioactive in situ hybridization studies is the identification of F4/80-positive macrophages expressing the erythropoietin gene in normal mouse bone marrow smears [9, 39]. These macrophages were nearly always in association with other cells surrounding the "central cell" as observed in "blood islands". Furthermore, of the approximately 10% F4/80-positive cells present in the normal mouse bone marrow, between 2% and 3%, or about 5×10^4 cells, express the erythropoietin gene.

Concluding Remarks

A subpopulation of the bone marrow macrophage can express the erythropoietin gene under normal steady-state conditions. In other words, erythropoietin gene expression occurs at the sites of erythropoiesis. This implies that the macrophage not only plays an "active" role in the hemopoietic cellular microenvironment, but also functions to regulate a biological system of which it is itself a part.

References

1. Jacobson LO, Goldwasser E, Fried W, Plzak LF (1957) The role of the kidney in erythropoiesis. Nature 179:633
2. Bondurant MC, Kourny MJ (1986) Anemia induces accumulation of erythropoietin mRNA in the kidney and liver. Mol Cell Biol 6:2731
3. Schuster SJ, Wildon JH, Erslev AJ, Caro J, (1987) Physiologic regulation and tissue localization of renal erythropoietin messenger RNA. Blood 70:316
4. Goldwasser E (1987) The molecular biology of erythropoietin and the expression of its gene. In: Rich IN (ed) Molecular and cellular aspects of erythropoietin and erythropoiesis. Springer, Berlin Heidelberg New York, pll (NATO ASI series, vol 8)
5. Caro J, Schuster S, Besarab A, Erslev AJ (1987) Renal biogenesis of erythropoietin. In: Rich IN (ed) Molecular and cellular aspects of erythropoietin and erythropoiesis. Springer, Berlin Heidelberg New York, p 329 (NATO ASI series, vol 8)
6. Nishida J, Hirai H, Kubota M, Lin F-K, Okabe T, Urabe A, Takaku F (1986) Detection of erythropoietin message in hypoxic mouse kidney. Jpn J Exp Med 56:321
7. Koury ST, Bondurant MC, Koury MJ (1988) Localization of erythropoietin synthesizing cells in murine kidneys by in situ hybridization. Blood 71:524
8. Lacombe C, Da Silva J-L, Bruneval P, Fournier J-G, Wendling F, Casadevall N, Camilleri J-P, Bariery J, Varet B, Tambourin P (1988) Peritubular cells are the site of erythropoietin synthesis in the murine hypoxic kidney. J Clin Invest 81:620
9. Rich IN, Vogt C, Pentz S (1988) Erythropoietin gene expression in vitro and in vivo detected by in situ hybridization. Blood Cells 14:505
10. Rudkin GT, Stollar BD (1977) High-resolution detection of DNA-RNA hybrids in situ by indirect immunofluorescence. Nature 265:472
11. Cheung SW, Tishler PV, Atkins L, Sengupta SK, Modest EJ, Forget BG (1977) Gene mapping by fluorescent in situ hybridization. Cell Biol Int Rep 1:255
12. Bauman JGJ, Wiegant J, Van Duijn P (1981) Cytochemical hybridization with fluorochrome-labeled RNA. I. Development of a method using nucleic acids bound to agarose beads as a model. J Histochem Cytochem 29:227
13. Bauman JGJ, Wiegant J, Van Duijn P (1981) Cytochemical hybridization with fluorochrome-labeled RNA. II. Applications. J Histochem Cytochem 29:238
14. Bauman JG, Wiegant J, Van Duijn P (1983) The development, using poly(Hg-U) in a model system, of a new method to visualize cytochemical hybridization in fluorescence microscopy. J Histochem Cytochem 31:571
15. Van der Ploeg M, Hopman AHN, Landegent JE, Raap AK, Wiegant J, Van Duijn P (1986) Non-radioactive in situ hybridization procedures using mercury- and acetylaminofluorene labelled probes. Acta Histochem Cytochem 19:701
16. Hopman AHN, Wiegant J, Van Duijn P (1987) Mercurated nucleic acid probes, a new principle for non-radioactive in situ hybridization. Exp Cell Res 169:357
17. Langer PR, Waldrop AA, Ward DC (1981) Enzymatic synthesis of biotin-labeled polynucleotides: novel nucleic acid affinity probes. Proc Natl Acad Sci USA 78:6633
18. Landegent JE, Jansen in de Wal N, Van Ommen GJB, Baas F, de Vijlder JJM, Van Duijn P, Van der Ploeg M (1985) Chromosomal localization of a unique gene by non-autoradiographic in situ hybridization. Nature 317:175
19. Singer RH, Ward DC (1982) Actin gene expression visualized in chicken muscle tissui culture by using in situ hybridization with a biotinated nucleotide analog. Proc Natl Acad Sci USA 79:7331
20. Brigati DJ, Myerson D, Leary JJ, Spalholz B, Travis SZ, Fong CKY, Hsiung GD, Ward DC (1983) Detection of viral genomes in cultured cells and paraffin-embedded tissue sections using biotin-labeled hybridization probes. Virology 126:32
21. Varndell IM, Polak JM, Sikri KL, Minth CD, Bloom SR, Dixon JE (1984) Visualisation of messenger RNA directing peptide synthesis by in situ hybridization using a novel single-stranded cDNA probe. Potential for the investigation of gene expression and endocrine cell activity. Histochem 8:597

22. Aksamit AJ, Mourrain P, Sever JL, Major EO (1985) Progressive multifocal leucoencephalopathy: investigation of three cases using in situ hybridization with JC virus biotinylated DNA probe. Ann Neurol 18:490
23. Milde K. Loening T (1986) Detection of papillomavirus DNA in oral papillomas and carcinomas: application of in situ hybridization with biotinylated HPV 16 probes. J Oral Pathol 15:292
24. Przepiorka D, Myerson D (1986) A single-step silver enhancement method permitting rapid diagnosis of cytomegalovirus infection in formalin-fixed, paraffin-embedded tissue sections by in situ hybridization and immunoperoxidase detection. J Histochem Cytochem 34:1731
25. Kaufman PH, Borstein J, Gordon AN, Adam E, Kaplan AL, Adler-storthz K (1987) Detection of human papillomavirus DNA in advanced epithelial ovarian carcinoma. Gynecol Oncol 27:340
26. Webster H, Lamperth L, Favilla JT, Lemka G, Tesin D, Manuelidis L (1987) Use of a biotinylated probe and in situ hybridization for light and electron microscopic localization of P_o mRNA in myelin-forming Schwann cells. Histochem 86:441
27. Hayashi S, Gillam IC, Delaney AD, Tener GM (1978) Acetylation of chromosome quashes of Drosophila melanogaster decreases the background in autoradiographs from hybridization with [^{125}I]-labelled RNA. J Histochem Cytochem 26:677
28. Rich IN (1987) Erythropoietin production by macrophages: cellular response to physiological oxygen tensions and detection of erythropoietin gene expression by in situ hybridization. In: Rich IN (ed) Molecular and cellular aspects of erythropoietin and erythropoiesis. Springer, Berlin Heidelberg New York, p 291 (NATO ASI series H, vol 8)
29. Kelemen E, Janossa M (1980) Macrophages are the first differentiated blood cells formed in the human embryonic liver. Exp Hematol 8:996
30. Gruber DF, Zucali JR, Mirand EA (1977) Identification of erythropoietin producing cells in fetal mouse liver cultures. Exp Hematol 12:825
31. Paul P, Rothmann SA, McMahon JT, Gordon AS (1984) Erythropoietin secretion by isolated rat Kupffer cells. Exp Hematol 12:825
32. Rich IN, Kubanek B (1985) The central role of the macrophage in hemopoietic microenvironmental regulation. In: Cronkite EP, Dainiak N, McCaffrey RP, Palek J, Quesenberry PJ (eds) Hematopoietic stem cell physiology. Liss, New York, p 283
33. Crocker P, Gordon S (1985) Isolation and characterization of resident stromal macrophages and hematopoietic cell clusters from mouse bone marrow. J Exp Med 162:993
34. De Jong JP, Nikkels PGJ, Piersma AH, Ploemacher RE (1987) Erythropoiesis and macrophage subsets in medullary and extramedullary sites. In: Rich IN (ed) Molecular and cellular aspects of erythropoietin and erythropoiesis. Springer, Berlin Heidelberg New York, p 237 (NATO ASI series H, vol 8)
35. Rich IN, Kubanek B (1982) Extrarenal erythropoietin production by macrophages. Blood 60:297
36. Rich IN (1986) A role of the macrophage in normal hemopoiesis. I. Functional capacity of bone-marrow-derived macrophages to release hemopoietic growth factors. Exp Hematol 14:738
37. Rich IN (1986) A role for the macrophage in normal hemopoiesis. II. Effect of varying physiological oxygen tensions on the release of hemopoietic growth factors from bone-marrow-derived macrophages in vitro. Exp Hematol 14:746
38. Rich IN (1988) The macrophage as a production site for hematopoietic regulator molecules: sensing and responding to normal and pathophysiological signals. Anticancer Res 8:1015
39. Vogt C, Pentz S, Rich IN. A role for the macrophage in normal hemopoiesis: III. In vitro and in vivo erythropoietin gene expression in macrophages detected by in situ hybridization. Exp Hematol (submitted for publication)
40. Ploem JS (1975) Reflection-contrast microscopy as a tool for investigation of the attachment of living cells to a glass surface. In: Furth RV (ed) Mononuclear phagocytes in immunity, infection and pathology. Blackwell, Oxford
41. Pentz S, Schulle H (1981) Revealing the adhesion mechanisms of cultured liver cells to glass surfaces during mitosis by reflection-contrast microscopy. Zeiss Information 25:41

Erythropoietin Synthesis in the Anemic Mouse Kidney as Observed by Morphological Techniques

P. Bruneval, J. L. Da Silva, C. Lacombe, J.-L. Salzmann,
P. Tambourin, B. Varet, J.-P. Camilleri, and J. Bariety

Erythropoietin (Epo) is the hormone regulating erythropoiesis in mammals. Although the major source of Epo in adults has been located in the kidneys [16], the nature of the renal Epo-producing cells is still debated. Immunofluorescence data [10] and glomerular [7] and mesangial [18] culture studies support a glomerular origin of the renal Epo-producing cells. On the other hand an extraglomerular origin of Epo-producing cells, i.e. tubular or interstitial, is suggested by studies based on renal tissue fractions [8, 25]. Furthermore, in a preliminary in situ hybridization study, we recently demonstrated that the renal Epo-producing cells were in a peritubular location [19]. Using the same techniques, these results were confirmed by other authors [17]. To better define the peritubular Epo-producing cells, we then investigated the nature of the renal peritubular cell population in the anemic and control mouse kidney, using electron microscopy and immunohistochemistry. The distribution of the Epo-producing cells within the kidney was assessed by morphometric analysis of the hybridized sections.

Materials and Methods

Induction of Epo Synthesis

It has been demonstrated that rapid accumulation of Epo mRNA in the murine kidney can be induced by anemia [4] or cobalt injection [3]. In order to increase the amount of kidney Epo mRNA and thus the in situ hybridization signal, ICFW mice were made profoundly anemic by a 6-Gy irradiation followed 24 h later by an intraperitoneal injection of phenylhydrazine (60 mg/kg body weight) [19]. Nine to 10 days later (hematocrit lower than 10%), mice were bled and their kidneys were removed. The kidneys were frozen in liquid nitrogen for in situ hybridization and poly(A)$^+$ RNA Northern blot analysis. A single characteristic band was detected at 1.8 kb by Northern blot analysis of the poly(A)$^+$ RNAs extracted from the anemic mouse kidney, whereas no signal was detected in normal mouse kidneys [19]. The Epo level in plasma of these anemic mice was between 6 and

10 IU/ml of serum by an in vitro bioassay using murine CFU-E derived colonies in plasma clot and by an in vivo bioassay using ^{59}Fe incorporation in polycythemic mice (normal: 20–30 mU/ml).

Probe

For in situ hybridization, a genomic probe was used [19]. This probe was a 243-bp *Pst*I-*Xho*II restriction fragment encompassing the second exon of the mouse Epo gene which was inserted at the *Pst*I and *Bam*HI sites of a pUC18 vector. A 265-bp Epo insert/pUC18 *Pst*I-*Eco*RI purified fragment was derived from this construct.

In Situ Hybridization

Five-micrometer-thick sections of unfixed frozen kidneys from six anemic and two control mice were prepared. They were fixed in 4% formaldehyde in 0.1 *M* phosphate buffer saline, pH 7.4, for 20 min and dehydrated in alcohols. The procedure for in situ hybridization has been previously described [6, 11, 19]. The tissue sections were immersed in HCl 0.2 *N* for 10 min. They were then incubated in 15 mg/ml proteinase K (protease XI, Sigma) in 20 m*M* Tris-HCl, pH 7.4, and 2 m*M* calcium chloride at 37 °C for 15 min. Tissue sections were then hybridized under a sealed coverslip for 24 h at 37 °C in 15 ml of a solution containing 50% deionized formamide, 10 m*M* Tris-HCl pH 7.4, 1 m*M* EDTA, 600 m*M* NaCl, 0.02% Ficoll, 0.02% polyvinylpyrrolidone, 0.02% bovine serum albumin, 10% dextran sulfate, 2 mg/ml yeast tRNA (Sigma), 400 mg/ml salmon sperm DNA (Sigma), 400 mg/ml herring sperm DNA (Sigma), 10 m*M* dithiothreitol, and 0.2 μg/ml of the radiolabeled probe denatured at 100 °C for 2 min. The probe was labeled by the random primer elongation method [9], with a commercially available kit (Amersham International, UK). Using ^{35}(S)dCTP (400 Ci/mmol), the specific activity of the probe was 2.10^8 cpm per μg of DNA.

The slides were then washed at room temperature with gentle agitation successively in 50% formamide-4 X SSC for 1 h, followed by two washes in 2 X SSC for 30 min and finally in 2 X SSC overnight. Sections were then dehydrated in alcohols and covered with Kodak NTB2 emulsion for autoradiography. After 10–12 days of exposure, the slides were developed in Kodak D19, fixed with Kodak A44, and stained with hematoxylin and eosin.

Three control procedures were performed to assess the specificity of the in situ hybridization labeling: (1) treatment of tissue sections with 50 μg/ml ribonuclease A (Type III, Sigma) in 2 X SSC for 30 min at 37 °C, rinsing for 30 min in 2 X SSC, followed by the hybridization with the Epo probe; (2) hybridization with a ^{35}S-labeled pUC18 vector without the Epo probe; (3) hybridization of nonanemic tissue kidney sections with the specific Epo probe.

Immunohistochemistry

Frozen kidney sections of a normal and an anemic mouse were fixed in cold acetone. Rabbit polyclonal anti-human Factor VIII-related (Willebrand) antigen antibody (DAKOPATTS, Copenhagen, Denmark) was used at a dilution of 1/100 in 0.1 *M* phosphate buffer saline pH 7.4. The indirect immunofluorescence technique was performed using a goat fluorescent anti-rabbit antibody (Institut Pasteur Production, France) at a dilution of 1/50. The monoclonal anti-F4/80 antibody, which recognizes a membrane antigen specific for murine monocyte-macrophage [15] was kindly provided by G. Milon (Institut Pasteur, Paris, France) and was used at a dilution of 1/32. Another anti-mouse monocyte-macrophage monoclonal antibody, M1/70 [14], was obtained commercially (Serotec, Realef, Paris, France), and used at a dilution of 1/20. These two antibodies were revealed using the peroxidase technique with peroxidase-conjugated anti-rat immunoglobulin antibody at a dilution of 1/200 (Biosys, Compiegne, France). Negative controls consisted of the omission of the specific antibodies. For positive controls, F 4/80 and M1/70 antibodies were tested in mouse liver and mouse spleen sections respectively.

Electron Microscopy

Small blocks of tissue from three anemic and one normal mouse kidney were fixed by immersion in 2.5% glutaraldehyde in PBS buffer 0.1 *M* (pH 7.4). After postfixation in 2% osmium tetroxide, the tissue samples were routinely processed for electron microscopy.

Image Analysis

An Epo probe-hybridized section from each of the six anemic mice was submitted to image analysis, as well as a ribonuclease-treated section and a nonanemic mouse kidney section. We used a computer vision image processor (NS 1500, Nachet-Vision, France), based upon the "mathematical morphology" theory [24]. Silver grain segmentation was easy at the magnification X100. Silver grains were isolated by "top hat" transformation to select them according to their size and contrast [20, 23]. Because of the silver grain image overlapping, their surface rather than their absolute number was calculated. For silver grain localization, the operator studied successively the cells of the glomeruli, the tubules, and the peritubular areas. The results were referred to a unit area of 100 μm^2. Fifteen measurements were performed for each cell type and histological localization. For statistical assessment, a Newman-Keuls test was performed in a one-way analysis of variance.

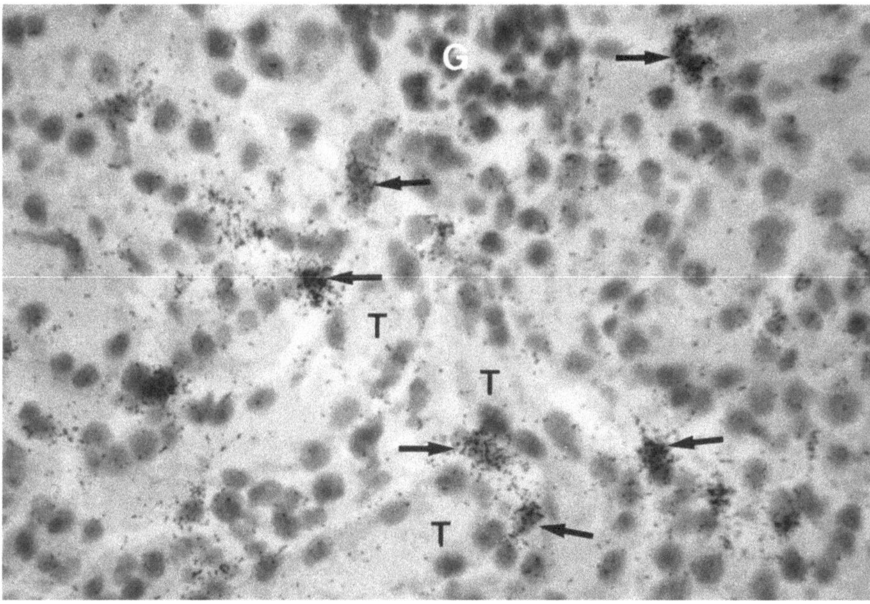

Fig. 1. In the anemic mouse kidney cortex, many positive cells (*arrows*) are detected in a peritubular location. Glomerulus (*G*) and tubules (*T*) are negative. In situ hybridization with Epo probe. H & E, X 300

Results

Renal specimens of all the mice, assessed by light microscopy in hematoxylin-eosin stained frozen sections, showed normal structure without any interstitial inflammatory infiltrates.

In situ hybridization of anemic mouse kidney sections detected an intense signal in many cells of the renal cortex and the outer medulla. The positive cells were clearly outside the glomeruli and outside the tubules, which were negative (Fig. 1). The labeled cells were in a peritubular location, some of them lining capillary lumina (Fig. 2). The nuclei of these cells were prominent between the tubules. Arteries and veins were negative. In the inner medulla no signal was detected. Similar results were obtained in all six kidneys. In control procedures, no positive cells could be detected in ribonuclease-treated sections or in sections hybridized with pUC18 plasmid. In kidney sections of the two normal mice, in situ hybridization with Epo probe failed to detect any signal.

The results of the image analysis of the six anemic and the two control mouse kidneys are expressed in Fig. 3. The silver grains counted on the glomeruli and the tubules of the control mouse kidneys represented the background. The silver grains counted on the glomeruli and the tubules of the anemic mouse kidneys were within

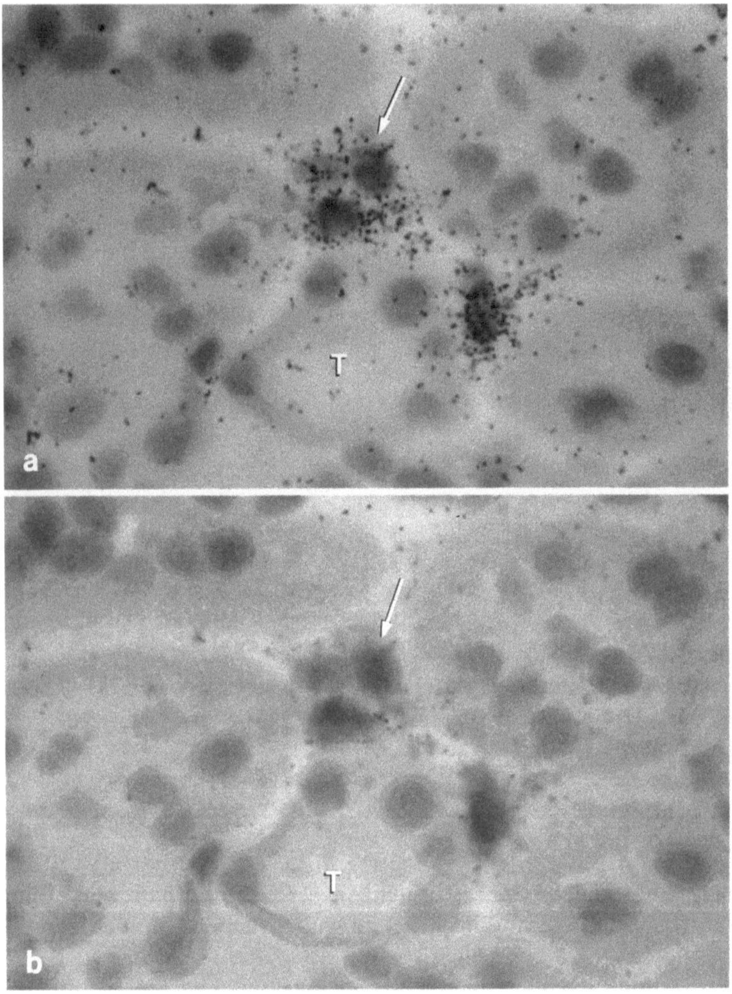

Fig. 2a, b. Higher magnifications clearly show that Epo-positive peritubular cells are lining a capillary vascular lumen (*arrow*). T, tubules. **a** Focused on silver grains at the level of autoradiographic emulsion; **b** focused on underlying renal tissue section. In situ hybridization with Epo probe. H & E, X 1200

the same range as the controls. Thus, they could be considered as background. The difference of grain areas on the labeled cells between the renal cortex and the outer medulla was significant in mice 1, 2, 5, and 6.

Immunohistochemical studies exhibited similar results in kidneys from both anemic and normal mice. With anti-human factor VIIIRAg (Willebrand antigen) antibody, a strong labeling was observed in endothelial cells lining peritubular capillaries and larger vessels in the renal cortex and the medulla (Fig. 4). Anti-

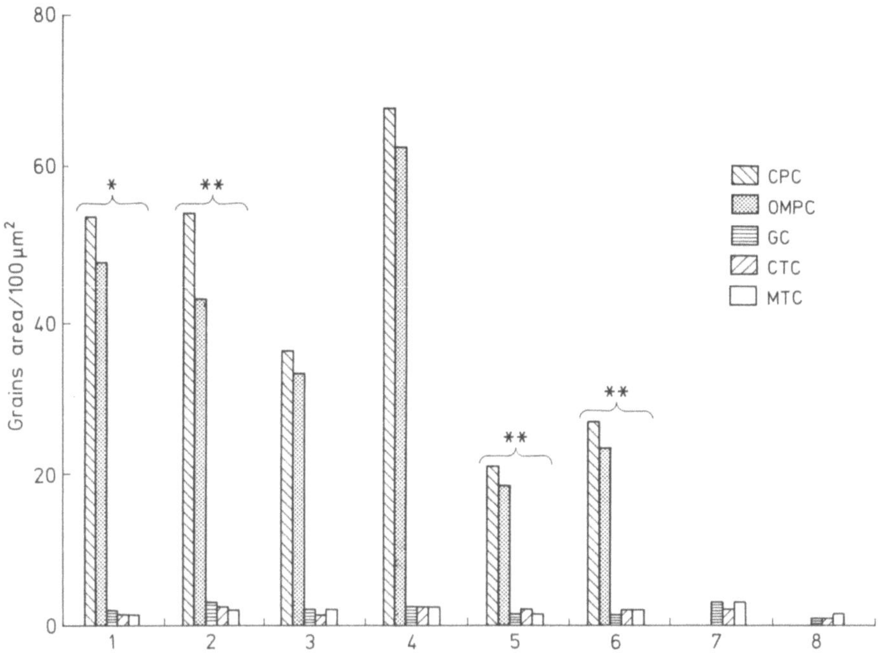

Fig. 3 Distribution of the areas of silver grains within the different structures of mouse kidney sections hybridized with Epo probe: anemic mouse kidneys (*1–6*), ribonuclease-treated anemic mouse kidney section (*7*), normal mouse kidney (*8*). *CPC,* cortical positive cells; *OMPC,* outer medullary positive cells; *GC,* glomerular cells; *CTC,* cortical tubular cells; *MTC* medullary tubular cells. *$p<0.05$; **$p<0.001$

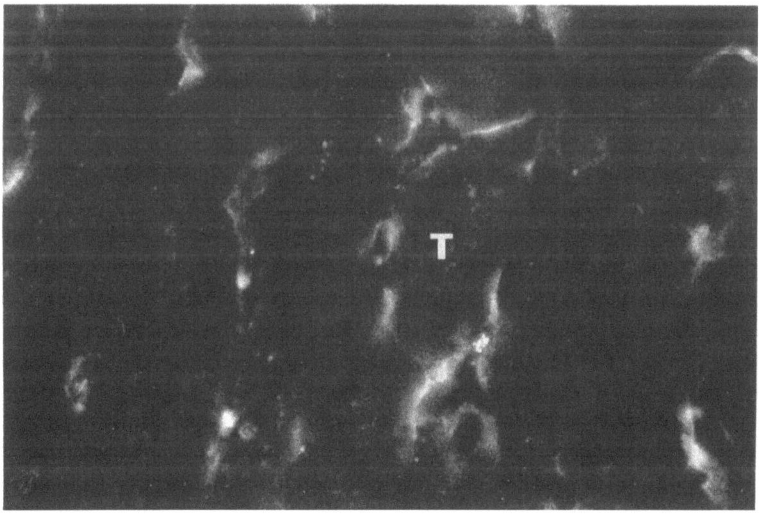

Fig. 4. Anti-human factor VIIIRAg (Willebrand antigen) antibody labels many endothelial cells around the tubules (*T*). Indirect Immunofluorescence in anemic mouse kidney section. X 300

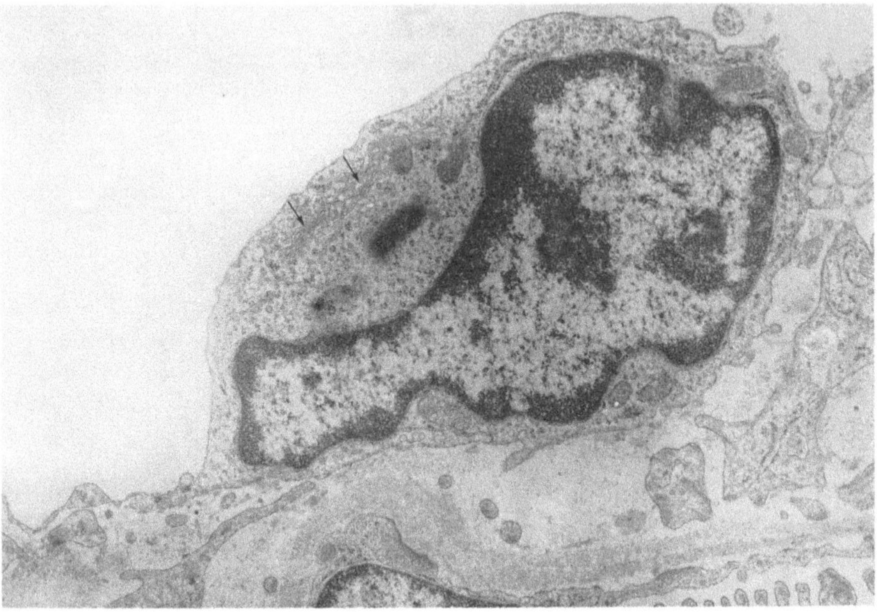

Fig. 5. Peritubular capillary endothelial cell exhibiting prominent Golgi apparatus (*arrows*), many free polyribosomes, and stands of rough endoplasmic reticulum. Electron microscopy in anemic mouse kidney. X 17000

mouse monocyte-macrophage antibodies F4/80 and M1/70 showed no labeling in most of the kidney sections or scanty labeled cells in rare sections, whereas they strongly labeled Kupffer cells in mouse liver and mononuclear cells in mouse red pulp spleen.

Ultrastructural study of the three anemic mouse kidneys showed that most of the peritubular cells in the renal cortex and the outer medulla were capillary endothelial cells. No inflammatory interstitial cells were observed. When compared with the normal mouse kidney, the peritubular capillary endothelial cells of the anemic mouse kidneys exhibited prominent rough and smooth reticulum, Golgi apparatus, and free polyribosomes (Fig. 5).

Discussion

These results demonstrate that under hypoxic conditions, the renal cells producing Epo in mice are in a peritubular location. Neither the glomeruli nor the tubules are involved in Epo mRNA synthesis in this animal model. However, given the sensitivity of the in situ hybridization technique, it cannot be ruled out that other renal cells are involved in Epo production under physiologic conditions. When the specificity of in situ hybridization is confirmed by controls, this technique demonstrates that a protein is definitely synthesized in a cell, and is not present in a cell by endocytosis. Immunohistochemistry cannot rule out endocytosis, which could explain earlier immunolocalization of Epo in the glomeruli [10].

In this study, image analysis confirms that the labeling is restricted to the peritubular cells; the grains counted on the glomeruli, the tubules, and the inner medulla and in the controls represent a low background. Furthermore, image analysis demonstrates a gradient of labeling beetween the cortex and the outer medulla. This suggests a gradient of Epo mRNA synthesis between the cortex and the outer medulla, the physiological significance of which is not clear. Image analysis is efficient to detect a heterogeneity of labeling between cells within the same section [21, 23, 27]. Given the resolution of the images obtained by in situ hybridization, the nature of the peritubular cells producing Epo mRNA has to be defined precisely by complementary techniques. As bone marrow macrophages have been implicated in Epo production [22], we first looked for macrophages in the mouse kidneys. Although no macrophages are observed in the interstitium of the normal human kidney [1], Hume and Gordon found macrophages around the mouse glomeruli and in the medulla [15]. However, using the same antibody F4/80 and another anti-mouse macrophage antibody (M1/70), we failed to detect any significant amount of macrophages in the mouse kidneys. Furthermore, the F4/80-labeled cells in the study of Hume and Gordon had not the topography of the Epo-producing cells. Second, another cell type, the renal Ia-positive dendritic cells [12], has to be discussed. The renal dendritic cells are mainly located in the renal cortex [12], and their distribution within the kidney is comparable to that of the Epo-producing cells. However, the renal dendritic cells reported by Hart and Fabre [12] are less numerous than the Epo-producing cells. Moreover, their existence in the kidney is controversial [1]. They would be endothelial cells [1], the bearing of Ia antigen on which is known [13]. Third, interstitial cells of the kidney were considered. They are a heterogeneous cell population [26]. Contrary to the cortical and outer medullary distribution of the Epo mRNA-producing cells, interstitial cells are mainly represented in the inner medulla. Finally, the peritubular capillary endothelial cells are candidates for Epo production because of the labeling of many cells in the same peritubular location by anti-human factor VIIIRAg (Willebrand antigen) an endothelial marker. Moreover, electron microscopy confirms that most of the peritubular cells in the normal and anemic mouse renal cortex are peritubular capillary endothelial cells [26]. When compared to the normal mouse kidney, the peritubular capillary endothelial cells of the anemic mouse kidney exhibit prominent cytoplasmic organelles consistent with an active cellular synthesis, suggesting that this cell type is actually involved in Epo synthesis.

The localization of Epo production in peritubular cells, probably capillary endothelial cells of the cortex and outer medulla, may have physiological implications. These cells are in close contact with the parts of the large renal tubules which are the major site of electrolyte reabsorption, associated with high energy and high oxygen consumption [2]. Furthermore, these parts of the large renal tubules are highly sensitive to hypoxia [5].

Summary

To characterize erythropoietin (Epo)-producing cells in the mouse kidney, in situ hybridization was performed in renal tissue sections using a radiolabeled genomic probe from the murine Epo gene. Epo production was dramatically increased by anemia induced by a 6-Gy irradiation and a 60-mg/kg body weight phenylhydrazine injection. This resulted in a 300-fold increase in serum Epo levels and in an intense characteristic band by Northern blot analysis of poly(A)$^+$ RNA in the kidney extracts. In situ hybridization detected a specific signal in many cells in the cortex and the outer medulla of the anemic mouse kidneys, whereas the inner medulla remained negative. The positive cells were clearly outside the glomeruli and outside the tubules. The Epo-producing cells were in a peritubular location. Immunohistochemistry and electron microscopy were conducted in parallel in normal and anemic mouse kidneys to assess the nature of these Epo-producing peritubular cells. They showed that most of the peritubular cells in the renal cortex and the outer medulla were peritubular capillary endothelial cells. Given these results, it is suggested that Epo-producing cells in the anemic mouse kidney are peritubular capillary endothelial cells. The distribution of the Epo-producing cells within the kidney was assessed by image analysis of the hybridized kidney sections. It showed that the cortical positive cells contained more silver grains than the medullary positive cells, suggesting a gradient of Epo mRNA synthesis betweeen the cortex and the medulla.

References

1. Alpers CE, Beckstead JH (1985) Monocyte/macrophage derived cells in normal and transplanted human kidneys. Clin Immunol Immunopathol 36: 129–140
2. Awquati QA, Chase HS Jr, Kleyman TR (1986) Cellular mechanisms of renal transport and metabolism. In: Brenner BM, Rector FC (eds) The kidney, 3rd edn. Saunders, Philadelphia, p 61
3. Beru N, MacDonald J, Lacombe C, Goldwasser E (1986) Expression of the erythropoietin gene. Mol Cell Biol 6: 2571–2575
4. Bondurant MC, Koury MJ (1986) Anemia induces accumulation of erythropoietin mRNA in the kidney and the liver. Mol Cell Biol 6: 2731–2733
5. Brezis M, Rosen S, Epstein FM (1986) Acute renal failure. In: Brenner BM, Rector FC (eds) The kidney, 3rd edn. Saunders, Philadelphia, p 735
6. Bruneval P, Fournier JG, Soubrier F, Belair MF, Da Silva JL, Guettier C, Pinet F, Tardivel I, Corvol P, Bariety J, Camilleri JP (1988) Detection and localization of renin messenger-RNA in human pathological tissues using in situ hybridization. Am J Pathol 131: 320–330
7. Burlington H, Cronkite EP, Reinke U, Zanjani ED (1972) Erythropoietin production in cultures of goat renal glomeruli. Proc Natl Acad Sci USA 69: 3547–3550
8. Caro J, Erslev AJ (1984) Biologic and immunologic erythropoietin in extracts from hypoxic whole rat kidneys and in their glomerular and tubular fractions. J Lab Clin Med 103: 922–931

9. Feinberg AP, Volgelstein B (1983) A technique for radiolabelling DNA restriction endonuclease fragments to high specific activity. Anal Biochem 132: 6–13
10. Fisher JW, Taylor G, Porteous DD (1965) Localization of erythropoietin in glomeruli of sheep kidney by fluorescent antibody technique. Nature 205: 611–612
11. Fournier JG, Tardieu M, Lebon P, Robain O, Ponsot G, Rozenblatt S, Bouteille M (1985) Detection of measles virus RNA in lymphocytes from peripheral blood and brain perivascular infiltrates of patient with subacute sclerosing panencephalitis. N Engl J Med 313: 910–915
12. Hart DNJ, Fabre W (1981) Major histocompatibility complex antigens in rat kidney, ureter, and bladder. Localization with monoclonal antibodies and demonstration of Ia-positive dendritic cells. Transplantation 31: 318–325
13. Hinglais N, Kazatchkine M, Charron DJ, Appay MD, Mandet C, Paing M, Bariety J (1984) Immunohistochemical study of Ia antigen in the normal and diseased human kidney. Kidney Int 25: 544–550
14. Ho MK, Springer TA (1982) Mac1 antigen: quantitative expression in macrophage populations and tissues, and immunofluorescent localization in spleen. J Immunol 128: 2281–2286
15. Hume DA, Gordon S (1983) Mononuclear phagocyte system of mouse defined by immunohystochemical localization of antigen F4/80. J Exp Med 157: 1704–1709
16. Jacobson LO, Goldwasser E, Fried W, Plzak L (1957) Role of the kidney in erythropoiesis. Nature 179: 633–634
17. Koury ST, Bondurant MC, Koury MJ (1988) Localization of erythropoietin synthesizing cells in murine kidneys by in situ hybridization. Blood 71: 524–527
18. Kurtz A, Jelkmann W, Sinowatz F, Bauer C (1983) Renal mesangial cell cultures as a model for study of erythropoietin production. Proc Natl Acad Sci USA 80: 4008–4011
19. Lacombe C, Da Silva JL, Bruneval P, Fournier JG, Wendling F, Casadevall N, Camilleri JP, Bariety J, Varet B, Tambourin P (1988) Peritubular capillary cells are the site of erythropoietin synthesis in the murine hypoxic kidney. J Clin Invest 81: 620–623
20. Meyer F (1977) Contrast feature extraction. In: Cherman JL (ed) Analyse quantitative des microstructures en sciences des materiaux, biologie et medecine, Rieder, Stuttgart, p 374
21. Poliard AM, Bernuau D, Tournier I, Legres LG, Schoevaert D, Feldmann G, Sala-Trepat JM (1986) Cellular analysis by in situ hybridization and immunoperoxidase of alfa-fetoprotein and albumin gene expression in rat liver during the perinatal period. J Cell Biol 103: 777–786
22. Rich IN, Heit W, Kubanek B (1982) Extrarenal erythropoietin production by macrophages. Blood 60: 1007–1018
23. Salzmann JL, Bernuau D, Poliard AM, Boussard C, Feldmann G (1986) An automatic method for counting silver grains in autohistoradiography: an application to in situ hybridization on rat liver cells. Acta Stereol 5: 273–278
24. Serra J (1972) Image analysis. Academic, London
25. Schuster SJ, Wilson JH, Erslev AJ, Caro J (1987) Physiologic regulation and tissue localization of renal erythropoietin messenger RNA. Blood 70: 316–318
26. Tischer CC, Madsen KM (1986) Anatomy of the kidney. In: Brenner BM, Rector FC (ed) The kidney, 3rd edn. Saunders, Philadelphia, p3
27. Tournier I, Bernuau D, Poliard AM, Schoevaert D, Feldmann G (1987) Detection of albumin mRNAs in rat liver gy in situ hybridization: usefulness of paraffin embedding and comparison of various fixation procedures. J Histochem Cytochem 35: 453–459

Tissue Hypoxia and the Production of Erythropoietin

H. Pagel, W. Jelkmann, and C. Weiss

Introduction

Tissue hypoxia is the major stimulus for the production of erythropoietin. The plasma level of the hormone may rise from a normal value of 5–20 mU/ml to 1000 mU/ml or more in severe anemia or during hypoxic hypoxia. The main functions of erythropoietin are to allow for compensation for the permanent loss of aged red blood cells and to increase erythropoiesis after hemorrhage.

Blood-borne erythropoietin is mainly of renal origin in adult mammals. Bilateral nephrectomy attenuates the erythropoietin response to hypoxia [15, 24, 32]. Erythropoietin activity has been demonstrated in extracts from hypoxic kidneys flushed free of blood [35]. Both erythropoietin and its mRNA are present mainly in the cortex of hypoxic kidneys. Perhaps peritubular capillary cells or interstitial mesenchymal cells are the site of the renal production of erythropoietin [39, 41]. As pointed out earlier, deoxygenation of blood in the kidney occurs mainly in the peritubular capillary network [34]. Therefore, O_2-sensitive tissue located in this area appears to be suited to detect decreases in the O_2 tension (pO_2) as well as in the O_2-carrying capacity of the blood.

Several factors have been implicated as positive messengers in the erythropoietin response to hypoxia, including prostanoids, adenosine and cyclic AMP (for references, see [19, 34]). At present, the variety of these putative mediators may mainly indicate that our understanding is still poor of the link between reduced O_2 supply to the tissues and the synthesis of erythropoietin in the kidney.

Moreover, we believe that a much more basic question still needs to be raised. As summarized in the feedback circuit shown in Fig. 1, it is generally assumed that the renal production of erythropoietin depends primarily on the pO_2 in the tissue of the kidney [23, 34]. In an attempt to evaluate the importance of the renal O_2-sensing mechanism, we carried out studies in which hypoxia was elicited in rats in different ways. The plasma erythropoietin level was studied: (a) at lowered arterial pO_2, (b) following the induction of anemia, and (c) at reduced blood flow to the kidneys. In this chapter, the results of these laboratory studies are reported with a view to the effects of hypoxia on the production of erythropoietin in humans.

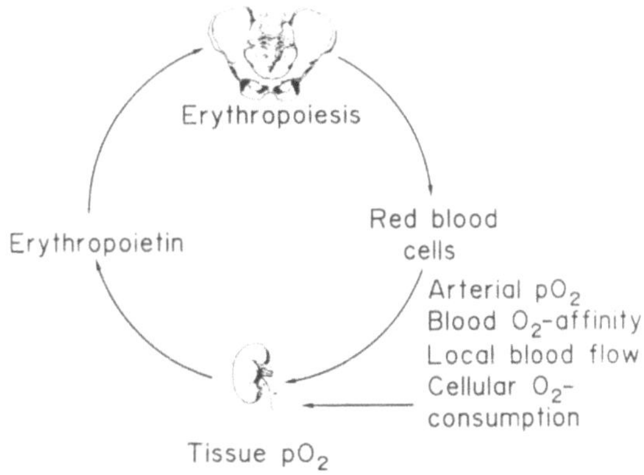

Fig. 1. Feedback control of erythropoiesis. Tissue hypoxia stimulates the production of erythropoietin, mainly in the kidneys. Augmented bone marrow erythropoiesis results in an increase in the concentration of red blood cells and, thus, the O_2 content of the blood

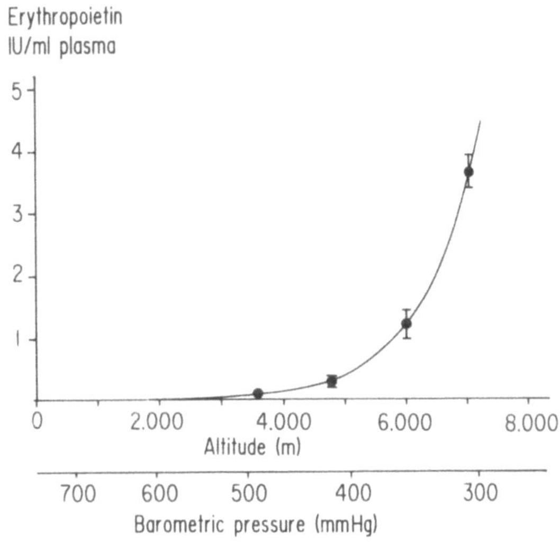

Fig. 2. Erythropoietin level in the plasma of male Sprague-Dawley rats after 16–18 h exposure to simulated altitude in a hypobaric chamber (mean ± SEM, $n = 4$–7). Modified from Jelkmann and Seidl [36]

Lowered Arterial O_2 Tension

Figure 2 illustrates the acute effect of lowering arterial pO_2 on the plasma level of erythropoietin in rats, as reported previously [36]. In brief, male Sprague-Dawley rats were exposed to different degrees of simulated altitude in a low pressure chamber. Erythropoietin was measured after 16–18 h exposure to hypoxia. The resulting plasma level of erythropoietin is shown as a function of the barometric pressure. It can be seen that the erythropoietin activity increased exponentially with the severity of hypoxia, reaching about 4 IU/ml plasma at 7000 m altitude [36]. Earlier studies had shown that plasma erythropoietin declines in rats after 18 h at continued exposure to hypoxia and eventually remains moderately elevated above normoxia values [6, 25, 33, 61]. A sustained rate of erythropoiesis is maintained in continuous hypoxia despite the decrease in the plasma erythropoietin level [12, 25].

A similar erythropoietin response occurs in humans following exposure to altitude. The concentration of erythropoietin increases for 1–2 days and then levels off to a value intermediate between sea level and the initial peak despite continued exposure to hypoxia [1, 18, 48, 50]. Using a sensitive radioimmunoassay for erythropoietin, Milledge and Cotes [48] have shown that the concentration of erythropoietin was indistinguishable from sea level normal in the blood of 10 lowlanders 3 weeks after the ascent to 4500 m. However, serum erythropoietin was still elevated above normal after 2–4 weeks at 6300 m. On descent to sea level, the concentration of erythropoietin decreased to the value in lowlanders within a day [48]. Scaro and Guidi [60] earlier found increased erythropoietin activity in only 10% of long-term altitude residents (4100 m) with hematocrits above 0.50.

Both sojourners and natives living at altitude exhibit an increased hematocrit and hemoglobin concentration. Bone marrow examinations of healthy natives of Morococha (4500 m) revealed extreme erythrocytic hyperplasia [47]. The benefits from the enhanced O_2-carrying capacity of the blood, however, are limited because of the increase in blood viscosity [13] and, therefore, cardiac work load. It was earlier assumed that the "optimal" hematocrit is 0.50–0.52 [65]. However, recent studies suggest that cerebral blood flow already decreases in man if the hematocrit exceeds 0.46 [64]. Chronic mountain sickness may develop when the hematocrit increases to very high values. If the persons remain at high altitude, insufficient peripheral blood flow, thrombosis and embolism, pulmonary hypertension and hypertrophy of the right lobe of the heart develops.

Freedman and Penington [22] earlier noted that patients with chronic respiratory failure and cyanosis tend to be polycythemic secondary to increased production of erythropoietin. However, more recent studies have shown that, unlike the response to hypoxia at altitude, there is no clear relationship between red cell mass and the arterial pO_2 or O_2 saturation in patients with chronic obstructive pulmonary disease. Neither has a relation been found between the occurrence of polycythemia and the level of bioactive [28] or immunoreactive [51, 71] erythropoietin. Vichinsky et al. [70] studied erythropoiesis in hypoxic patients suffering from cystic fibrosis. The hemoglobin concentration and erythropoietin level in the victims were not elevated. Moreover, one third of the patients were anemic [70]. Note that hypercapnia is frequently associated with chronic respiratory failure. There is some evidence that the synthesis of erythropoietin depends on pH (for references, see [34]). Low plasma erythropoietin levels were observed in hypercapnic anemic rats [49]. On the other hand, in the study by Guidet et al. [28] the pCO_2 was significantly

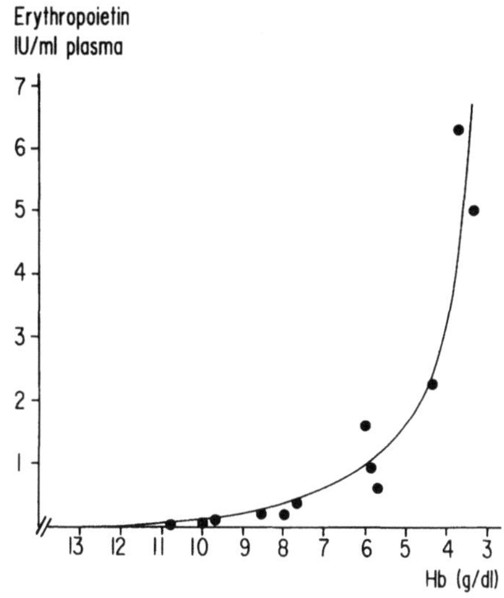

Fig. 3. Erythropoietin level in the plasma of male Sprague-Dawley rats 17–18 h after isovolemic anemia was induced by hemodilution. Modified from Jelkmann and Seidl [36] and Pagel et al. [55]

higher in the blood of the polycythemic group of patients with chronic obstructive pulmonary disease than in the polycythemic group.

In addition, erythrocytosis secondary to low systemic arterial pO_2 occurs in patients with cyanotic congenital heart disease. The concentration of erythropoietin in the blood of the patients has been found to vary considerably. While Tyndall et al. [67] and Gidding et al. [27] have reported high erythropoietin levels (>30 mU/ml) in patients with low arterial pO_2 and low arterial O_2 saturation, other investigators failed to demonstrate a correlation of the erythropoietin level with the hemoglobin concentration, hematocrit, arterial pO_2 or arterial O_2 saturation [29, 37]. The proportion of patients with abnormally high plasma erythropoietin levels in these studies ranged from 76 % [37] to 11% [29]. The reason for the wide variability in the plasma erythropoietin level in patients with cyanotic congenital heart disease is not known. Jindal et al. [37] have proposed that a new steady state could be reached in the patients with low plasma erythropoietin. In other words, the reduced arterial O_2 saturation is perhaps compensated by the increase in the O_2-carrying capacity of the blood.

Anemic Hypoxia

Figure 3 illustrates the effect of acute anemia on the plasma level of erythropoietin in rats, as reported previously [36, 55]. In brief, anemia of differing severity was induced in male Sprague-Dawley rats by hemodilution. As described by Lechermann and Jelkmann [43], defined blood portions were withdrawn through a catheter in a carotid artery. The blood was immediately replaced by equal volumes of heparinized plasma which was freshly prepared from normal Spraque-Dawley rats. The plasma erythropoietin activity is shown as a function of the hemoglobin concentration in the blood 17–18 h after the exchange transfusion. There is an exponential relationship between the erythropoietin concentration and the degree of anemia. Plasma erythropoietin was about 6 IU/ml when the hemoglobin concentration was reduced to 25 % of normal.

In humans without renal disease, a similar inverse relationship exists between the plasma erythropoietin level and the hemoglobin concentration [2, 9] or the hematocrit [16, 69]. Very low erythropoietin levels (<5 mU/ml) have been determined in patients with polycythemia vera [8, 10, 16, 26, 73]. In anemia, the plasma level of erythropoietin may increase by 3 orders of magnitude above the normal value of 5–20 mU/ml. Erslev et al. [16, 17] have noted an exponential (or semilogarithmic) relationship between the erythropoietin concentration and the hematocrit in nonuremic patients independently of the type of anemia. However, there is some evidence that the level of erythropoietin is not only dependent on the degree of anemia. Reduced levels of erythropoietin may be found in chronic diseases of inflammation or malignancy (for references, see [38]). On the other hand, it has been suspected that the plasma level of erythropoietin is more elevated in patients with severe bone marrow insufficiency than in patients with active erythropoiesis at similar degrees of anemia. Indeed, plasma erythropoietin is extremly high in patients with hypoplastic anemias [9, 30, 46, 54, 56]. It is not clear whether the increase in plasma erythropoietin results from diminished marrow utilization of the hormone [9] or whether a feedback regulation mechanism operates between the proliferative activity of erythrocytic progenitors and the synthesis of erythropoietin in the kidney in addition to the effects of tissue hypoxia on the production of erythropoietin [4, 46].

Anemia is an almost inevitable complication of chronic renal failure. The anemia is generally normochronic and normocytic. Several factors may contribute to the anemia, including a relative or absolute erythropoietin deficiency, bleeding, a shortened red cell life span, and toxic inhibition of erythropoiesis (for references, see [59]). Although some endocrine function may be maintained, damaged kidneys are incapable of increasing the blood level of erythropoietin sufficiently to restore red cell mass. In the anemia of renal failure the erythropoietin bioactivity in blood is considerably less than it is in other types of anemia [11, 16, 42, 58]. Recent radioimmunological measurements have confirmed this observation. In addition, the usual negative correlation between the concentration of erythropoietin in blood and the hematocrit or hemoglobin level has been missed in some of the reports on the anemia of chronic renal failure [45, 53, 56] though not in all [68]. Patients have been studied with end stage renal disease of different etiology, including chronic glomerulonephritis, diabetic nephropathy, chronic pyelonephritis and interstitial nephritis. De Klerk et al. [11] have noted that in dialysis patients the dependence on transfusion therapy was not associated with the underlying renal disease. However, in predialysis patients with chronic glomerulonephritis, the blood level of erythropoietin and hemoglobin were inversely correlated, whereas in predialysis patients with chronic nonglomerular disease no such correlation existed. This

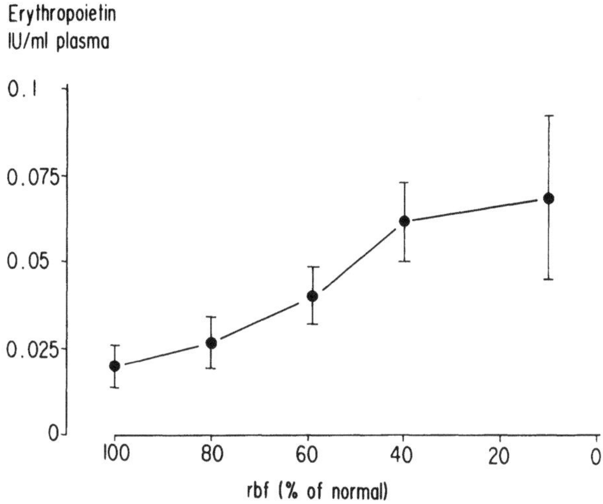

Fig. 4. Erythropoietin level in the plasma of male Sprague-Dawley rats 18–20 h after renal blood flow (*rbf*) was reduced bilaterally by the application of silver clamps (mean ± SEM, n = 3–5). Modified from Pagel et al. [55]

observation is of interest in view of the recent localization of erythropoietin mRNA in peritubular capillary cells in the kidney cortex [39, 41].

Reduced Renal Blood Flow

Figure 4 shows the effect of an acute lowering of the O_2 supply to the kidneys alone. As reported recently, in these studies the renal blood flow in rats was reduced bilaterally by the application of silver clamps [55]. The degree of the reduction of renal blood flow was adjusted by clamps of different diameters. Renal blood flow was measured by means of an electromagnetic flowmeter. Blood for the bioassay of erythropoietin was sampled 18–20 h after the renal arteries were clamped. A linear relationship was found between the erythropoietin level and the reduction of the renal blood flow (Fig. 4). In addition, the plasma level of erythropoietin did not exceed 0.07 IU/ml, even when the renal blood flow was reduced to 10% of normal. These findings indicate that, in contrast to a reduced whole body O_2 offer, a reduction of the blood flow to the kidneys alone is a minor stimulus for the production of erythropoietin. Previously, some authors have noted an increase in the level of erythropoietin in the blood of experimental animals with constricted renal arteries [20, 21, 52, 62], while other investigators have reported negative results [7, 74].

A reduction of the renal blood flow results in a lowered tubular sodium load. In turn, a lowered sodium load leads to a decrease in the O_2 demand of the kidney

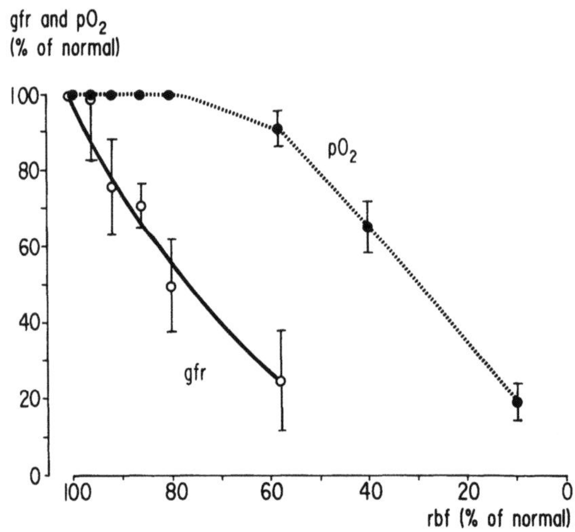

Fig. 5. Effects of lowering renal blood flow (*rbf*) on the O_2 tension (pO_2) in renal venous blood (mean ± SEM, $n = 10$) and on the glomerular filtration rate (*gfr;* mean ± SEM, $n = 5$) in male Sprague-Dawley rats

[40, 66]. As noted earlier, the production of erythropoietin is thought to depend on the pO_2 in the kidney tissue, which is determined by the ratio of renal O_2 supply to renal O_2 demand. Therefore, we studied whether a constriction of the renal artery leads to hypoxia in the kidney. The pO_2 of mixed renal venous blood was measured by means of a polarographic needle probe [72]. As shown in Fig. 5, the pO_2 of the renal venous blood began to decrease gradually only if the blood flow was reduced below 80% of normal. The renal venous pO_2 was less than 10 mmHg when the renal blood flow was reduced to 10% of normal. Thus, a reduction in renal blood flow results in a significant lowering of the pO_2 in the kidney, despite the concomitant decrease in glomerular filtration (Fig. 5), sodium load and O_2 demand.

With regard to human physiology, it seems unlikely that adaptational changes in renal blood flow exert significant effects on the rate of the synthesis of erythropoietin. Bourgoignie et al. [5] noted a slight increase in the plasma erythropoietin level in 60% of 18 hypertensive patients with severe renal arterial stenosis. Surgical corrections of the renal arterial lesion lowered the erythropoietin level. None of the patients was polycythemic. Indeed, renal arterial stenosis is very rarely associated with erythrocytosis [3, 31, 44, 63].

Summary and Conclusions

A reduction of the whole body O_2 offer greatly stimulates the production of erythropoietin. It is reasonable to assume that blood–borne erythropoietin is

Table 1. Diseases associated with an inappropriate production of erythropoietin and clinical manifestations

A.	Erythrocytosis due to overproduction of erythropoietin
	Chronic mountain sickness
	Chronic respiratory diseases
	Cyanotic heart diseases
	Hemoglobinopathies with increased O_2 affinity
	Renal arterial stenosis (erythrocytosis not common)
	Renal cysts
	Erythropoietin-producing neoplasms
B.	Anemia due to insufficient production of erythropoietin
	Chronic renal failure

mainly of renal origin. On the other hand, the level of erythropoietin in blood increases little when the O_2 supply to the kidneys alone is lowered by reducing renal blood flow. Thus, the production of erythropoietin seems to depend only partly on the O_2 supply to the kidneys. Future studies may clarify the importance of extrarenal O_2-sensitive mechanisms which could influence the renal production of erythropoietin via nervous or humoral factors.

The erythropoietin response to anemia implies that the arterial pO_2 is not the primary determinant of the production of erythropoietin, because the arterial pO_2 is not lowered in anemia. Instead the relevant O_2-sensitive cells in control of the hormone must be located at the venous side of the microcirculation. Hence, the O_2 content of the blood is the important parameter which is determined both by the O_2–carrying capacity and by the pO_2. In addition, the O_2 affinity and the rate of flow of the blood have some effects on the pO_2 of the tissues. In recalling the feedback circuit shown in Fig. 1, the following erythropoietin-dependent disturbances in erythropoiesis can be deduced (Table 1).

Secondary erythrocytosis is due to an overproduction of erythropoietin. Blood viscosity is increased. Venous thrombosis and heart failure may develop. Secondary erythrocytosis is a manifestation of chronic mountain sickness. In addition, it may occur in cardiopulmonary diseases and hemoglobinopathies leading to impaired O_2 supply to the tissues, in renal artery stenosis, and in association with erythropoietin-producing neoplasms.

Anemia due to an insufficient production of erythropoietin seems to occur in renal failure only. Here, the use of recombinant human erythropoietin to stimulate erythropoiesis may prevent the need for blood transfusions with their risks of infections and iron overload.

References

1. Abbrecht PH, Littell JK (1972) Plasma erythropoietin in men and mice during acclimatization to different altitudes. J Appl Physiol 32: 54–58
2. Alexanian R (1973) Erythropoietin excretion in bone marrow failure and hemolytic anemia. J Lab Clin Med 82: 438–445
3. Bacon BR, Rothman SA, Ricanati ES, Rashad FA (1980) Renal artery stenosis with erythrocytosis after renal transplantation. Arch Intern Med 140: 1206–1211
4. Barceló AC, Bozzini CE (1982) Erythropoietin formation during hypoxia in mice with impaired responsiveness to erythropoietin induced by irradiation or 5-fluorouracil injection. Experientia 38: 504–505
5. Bourgoignie JJ, Gallagher NI, Perry MH, Kurz L, Warnecke MA, Donati RM (1968) Renin and erythropoietin in normotensive and in hypertensive patients. J Lab Clin Med 71: 523–536
6. Caro J, Erslev AJ (1984) Biologic and immunologic erythropoietin in extracts from hypoxic whole rat kidneys and in their glomerular and tubular fractions. J Lab Clin Med 103: 922–931
7. Cooper GW, Nocenti MR (1961) Unilateral renal ischemia and erythropoietin. Proc Soc Exp Biol Med 108: 546–549
8. Cotes PM, Doré CJ, Liu Yin JA, Lewis SM, Messinezy M, Pearson TC, Reid C (1986) Determination of serum immunoreactive erythropoietin in the investigation of erythrocytosis. N Engl J Med 315: 283–287
9. De Klerk G, Rosengarten PCJ, Vet RJWM, Goudsmit R (1981) Serum erythropoietin (ESF) titers in anemia. Blood 58: 1164–1170
10. De Klerk G, Rosengarten PCJ, Vet RJWM, Goudsmit R (1981) Serum erythropoietin (ESF) titers in polycythemia. Blood 58: 1171–1174
11. De Klerk G, Wilmink JM, Rosengarten PCJ, Vet RJWM, Goudsmit R (1982) Serum erythropoietin (ESF) titers in anemia of chronic renal failure. J Lab Clin Med 100: 720–734
12. Dunn CDR, Smith LN, Leonard JI, Andrews RB, Lange RD (1980) Animal & computer investigations into the murine erythroid response to chronic hypoxia. Exp Hematol 8 [Suppl 8]: 259–279
13. Erslev AJ, Caro J (1984) Secondary polycythemia: a boon or a burden? Blood Cells 10: 177–191
14. Erslev AJ, Caro J (1984) Pure erythrocytosis classified according to erythropoietin titers. Am J Med 76: 57–61
15. Erslev AJ, Caro J, Kansu E, Silver R (1980) Renal and extrarenal erythropoietin production in anaemic rats. Br J Haematol 45: 65–72
16. Erslev AJ, Caro J, Miller O, Silver R (1980) Plasma erythropoietin in health and disease. Ann Clin Lab Sci 10: 250–257
17. Erslev AJ, Wilson J, Caro J (1987) Erythropoietin titers in anemic, nonuremic patients. J Lab Clin Med 109: 429–433
18. Faura J, Ramos J, Reynafarje C, English E, Finne P, Finch CA (1969) Effect of altitude on erythropoiesis. Blood 33: 668–676
19. Fisher JW (1988) Pharmacologic modulation of erythropoietin production. Annu Rev Pharmacol Toxicol 28: 101–122
20. Fisher JW, Samuels AI (1967) Relationship between renal blood flow and erythropoietin production in dogs. Proc Soc Exp Biol Med 125: 482–485
21. Fisher JW, Schofield R, Porteous DD (1965) Effects of renal hypoxia on erythropoietin production. Br J Haematol 11: 382–388
22. Freedman BJ, Penington DG (1963) Erythrocytosis in emphysema. Br J Haematol 9: 425–430
23. Fried W (1975) Erythropoietin and the kidney, Nephron 15: 327–349
24. Fried W, Kilbridge T, Krantz S, McDonald TP, Lange RD (1969) Studies on extrarenal erythropoietin. J Lab Clin Med 73: 244–248

25. Fried W, Johnson C, Heller P (1970) Observations on regulation of erythropoiesis during prolonged periods of hypoxia. Blood 36: 607–616
26. Garcia JF, Ebbe SN, Hollander L, Cutting HO, Miller ME, Cronkite EP (1982) Radioimmunoassay of erythropoietin: circulating levels in normal and polycythemic human beings. J Lab Clin Med 99: 624–635
27. Gidding SS, Stockman JA (1988) Erythropoietin in cyanotic heart disease. Am Heart J 116: 128–132
28. Guidet B, Offenstadt G, Boffa G, Najman A, Baillou C, Hatzfeld C, Amstutz P (1987) Polycythemia in chronic obstructive pulmonary disease. Chest 92: 867–870
29. Hågå P, Cotes PM, Till JA, Minty BD, Shinebourne EA (1987) Serum immunoreactive erythropoietin in children with cyanotic and acyanotic congenital heart disease. Blood 70: 822–826
30. Hammond D, Shore N, Movassaghi N (1968) Production, utilization and excretion of erythropoietin: I. Chronic anemias. II. Aplastic crisis. III. Erythropoietic effects of normal plasma. Ann NY Acad Sci 149: 516–527
31. Hudgson P, Pearce JMS, Yeates WK (1967) Renal artery stenosis with hypertension and high haematocrit. Br Med J 1: 18–21
32. Jacobson LO, Marks EK, Gaston EO, Goldwasser E (1959) Studies on erythropoiesis. XI. Reticulocyte response of transfusion-induced polycythemic mice to anemic plasma from nephrectomized mice and to plasma from nephrectomized rats exposed to low oxygen. Blood 14: 635–643
33. Jelkmann W (1982) Temporal pattern of erythropoietin titers in kidney tissue during hypoxic hypoxia. Pflügers Arch 393: 88–91
34. Jelkmann W (1986) Renal erythropoietin: properties and production. Rev Physiol Biochem Pharmacol 104: 139–215
35. Jelkmann W, Bauer C (1981) Demonstration of high levels of erythropoietin in rat kidney following hypoxic hypoxia. Pflügers Arch 392: 34–39
36. Jelkmann W, Seidl J (1987) Dependence of erythropoietin production on blood oxygen affinity and hemoglobin concentration in rats. Biomed Biochim Acta 46: S 304–S 308
37. Jindal SK, Gupta B, Mohanty D, Das KC, Bidwai PS, Wahi PL (1978) Study of erythropoiesis, erythropoietin and haematological adjustments in congenital cyanotic heart disease. Indian J Med Res 67: 1019–1028
38. Johannsen H, Gross AJ, Jelkmann W (1989) Erythropoietin production in malignancy. In: Jelkmann W, Gross AJ (eds) Erythropoietin. Springer-Verlag Berlin Heidelberg New York, pp 80–91
39. Koury ST, Bondurant MC, Koury MJ (1988) Localization of erythropoietin synthesizing cells in murine kidneys by in situ hybridization. Blood 71: 524–527
40. Kramer K, Deetjen P (1960) Beziehungen des O_2–Verbrauchs der Niere zu Durchblutung und Glomerulusfiltrat bei Änderung des arteriellen Druckes. Pflügers Arch 271: 782–796
41. Lacombe C, Da Silva JL, Bruneval P, Fournier JG, Wendling F, Casadevall N, Camilleri JP, Bariety J, Varet B, Tambourin P (1988) Peritubular cells are the site of erythropoietin synthesis in the murine hypoxic kidney. J Clin Invest 81: 620–623
42. Lange RD, Gallagher NI (1962) Clinical and experimental observations on the relationship of the kidney to erythropoietin production. In: Jacobson L, Doyle M (eds) Erythropoiesis. Grune and Stratton, New York, pp 361–373
43. Lechermann B, Jelkmann W (1985) Erythropoietin production in normoxic and hypoxic rats with increased blood O_2 affinity. Respir Physiol 60: 1–8
44. Luke RG, Kennedy AC, Barr Stirling WB, McDonald GA (1965) Renal artery stenosis, hypertension, and polycythaemia. Br Med J 1: 164–166
45. McGonigle RJS, Wallin JD, Shadduck RK, Fisher JW (1984) Erythropoietin deficiency and inhibition of erythropoiesis in renal insufficiency. Kidney Int 25: 437–444
46. McGonigle RJS, Ohene-Frempong K, Lewy JE, Fisher JW (1985) Erythropoietin response to anaemia in children with sickle cell disease and Fanconi's hypoproliferative anaemia. Acta Haematol 74: 6–9

47. Merino CF, Reynafarje C (1952) Bone marrow studies in the polycythemia of high altitudes. J Lab Clin Med 142: 637–647
48. Milledge JS, Cotes PM (1985) Serum erythropoietin in humans at high altitude and its relation to plasma renin. J Appl Physiol 59: 360–364
49. Miller ME, Howard D (1979) Modulation of erythropoietin concentrations by manipulation of hypercarbia. Blood Cells 5: 389–403
50. Miller ME, Rørth M, Parving HH, Howard D, Reddington I, Valeri CR, Stohlman F (1973) pH effect on erythropoietin response to hypoxia. N Engl J Med 288: 706–710
51. Miller ME, Garcia JF, Cohen RA, Cronkite EP, Moccia G, Acevedo J (1981) Diurnal levels of immunoreactive erythropoietin in normal subjects and subjects with chronic lung disease. Br J Haematol 49: 189–200
52. Mujovic VM, Fisher JW (1974) The effects of indomethacin on erythropoietin production in dogs following renal artery constriction. I. The possible role of prostaglandins in the generation of erythropoietin by the kidney. J Pharmacol Exp Ther 191: 575–580
53. Naets JP, Garcia JF, Tousaaint C, Buset M, Waks D (1986) Radioimmunoassay of erythropoietin in chronic uraemia or anephric patients. Scand J Haematol 37: 390–394
54. Napier JAF, Dunn CDR, Ford TW, Price V (1977) Pathophysiological changes in serum erythropoiesis stimulating activity. Br J Haematol 35: 403–409
55. Pagel H, Jelkmann W, Weiss C (1988) A comparison of the effects of renal artery constriction and anemia on the production of erythropoietin. Pflügers Arch 413: 62–66
56. Pavlović-Kentera V, Milenković P, Ruvidić R, Jovanović V, Biljanović-Paunović L (1979) Erythropoietin in aplastic anemia. Blut 39: 345–350
57. Pavlović-Kentera V, Clemons GK, Djukanović L, Biljanocić-Paunović L (1987) Erythropoietin and anemia in chronic renal failure. Exp Hematol 15: 785–789
58. Penington DG (1961) The role of the erythropoietic hormone in anaemia. Lancet i: 301–306
59. Powell JS, Adamson JW (1985) Hematopoiesis and the kidney. In: Seldin DW, Giebisch G (eds) The kidney: physiology and pathophysiology. Raven, New York, pp 847–866
60. Scaro JL, Guidi EE (1970) Relationship between plasma erythropoietin activity and hematocrit ratio in high altitude residents. Acta Physiol Latinoam 20: 103–105
61. Schooley JC, Mahlmann LJ (1975) Hypoxia and the initiation of erythropoietin production. Blood Cells 1: 429–448
62. Takaku F, Hirashima K, Nakao K (1962) Studies on the mechanism of erythropoietin production. I. Effect of unilateral constriction of the renal artery. J Lab Clin Med 59: 815–820
63. Tarazi RC, Frohlich ED, Dustan HP, Gifford RW, Page IH (1966) Hypertension and high hematocrit. Am J Cardiol 18: 855–858
64. Thomas DJ, Du Boulay GH, Marshall J, Pearson TC, Ross Russell RW, Symon L, Wetherley-Mein G, Zilkha E (1977) Effect of haematocrit on cerebral blood-flow in man. Lancet ii: 941–943
65. Thorling EB, Erslev AJ (1968) The "tissue" tension of oxygen and its relation to hematocrit and erythropoiesis. Blood 31: 332–343
66. Thurau K (1961) Renal Na reabsorption and O_2 uptake in dogs during hypoxia and hydrochlorothiazide infusion. Proc Soc Exp Biol Med 106: 714–717
67. Tyndall MR, Teitel DF, Lutin WA, Clemons GK, Dallman PR (1987) Serum erythropoietin levels in patients with congenital heart disease. J Pediatr 110: 538–544
68. Urabe A, Saito T, Fukamachi H, Kubota M, Takaku F (1987) Serum erythropoietin titers in the anemia of chronic renal failure and other hematological states. Int J Cell Cloning 5: 202–208
69. Van Dyke DC, Layrisse M, Lawrence JH, Garcia JF, Pollycove M (1961) Relation between severity of anemia and erythropoietin titer in human beings. Blood 18: 187–201
70. Vichinsky EP, Pennathur-Das R, Nickerson B, Minor M, Kleman K, Higashino S, Lubin B (1984) Inadequate erythroid response to hypoxia in cystic fibrosis. J Pediatr 105: 15–21
71. Wedzicha JA, Cotes PM, Empey DW, Newland AC, Royston JP, Tam RC (1985) Serum immunoreactive erythropoietin in hypoxic lung disease with and without polycythaemia. Clin Sci 69: 413–422

72. Weiss C, Fleckenstein W (1986) Local tissue pO_2 measured with "thick" needle probes. Funktionsanal Biol Syst 15: 155–166
73. Zaroulis CG, Hoffman BJ, Kourides IA (1981) Serum concentrations of erythropoietin measured by radioimmunoassay in hematologic disorders and chronic renal failure. Am J Hematol 11: 85–92
74. Živný J, Kolc J, Málek P, Neuwirt J (1972) Renal ischaemia, hypoxic hypoxia and erythropoietin production. Scand J Haematol 9: 470–476

Early Anemia in Mammals

S. Halvorsen, M. Hellebostad, P. Holter, P. Hågå, A. Meberg, and T. Sanengen

Most data indicate that the basic hypoxia-erythropoietin mechanism operates in fetal life and also postnatally. This means that erythropoietin increases following hypoxia irrespective of the production site of the hormone and decreases when there is a surplus of oxygen-carrying capacity. There are, however, several studies indicating that regulation of erythropoiesis in the neonatal mammal differs from that in the adult [1, 2]. Erythropoiesis in the perinatal period is not a steady-state condition, it is constantly changing. This must be taken into consideration both regarding the experimental design and the conclusions that can be drawn from the studies.

In order to learn more about the regulatory mechanisms in this age period, we used traditional approaches. First we recorded what went on in different species. Second we observed whether it was possible to suppress erythropoiesis and erythropoietin production either by blood transfusion or by iron supplementation. Third, we studied the effects of hypoxia, anemic or hypobaric, and fourth, we tried to characterize the high erythropoiesis-stimulating activity found in the plasma of mice at the time of weaning, that is, 20 days. The fifth approach was to study the effect of possible known erythropoietic candidates on erythropoiesis in the actual age period.

Early Anemia and Erythropoietin

Our group has studied erythropoiesis in full-term and preterm infants and in young mice, rats, and rabbits. They all develop a fall in hemoglobin concentration postnatally, early anemia. The anemia is moderate in the full-term human infant, but may be severe in preterm infants and in the other species studied. Both in mice, rats, and rabbits the nadir of the PCV levels is at the time of weaning [3]. In the human it is not easy to say when weaning occurs. Erythropoietin measured by an in vitro method increases markedly in the three animal species studied, with the highest levels at or after the nadir of the anemia [3]. In the preterm infant the levels are only moderately elevated [4]. With RIA Hellebostad et al. [5] found in full-term babies, low concentrations of erythropoietin at the age of 2 months and normal adult levels from the age of 3 months. Other workers have found only slight elevation of erythropoietin in preterm infants [6, 7], suggesting a lack of erythropoietin in these infants. This finding and the fact that prematurity in itself is a pathological condition suggest that the cause of early anemia is different in premature infants compared with other mammals.

In young rabbits during early anemia, oxygen-carrying capacity did not fall due to rise in 2,3-diphosphoglycerate (DPG). The rise in 2,3-DPG was the same when the early anemia was abolished following iron therapy, suggesting that the rise in 2,3-DPG is a preprogrammed event [8, 9]. In young mice erythropoietic stimulating factor (ESF) concentrations increased further after PCV started to rise and remained relatively high, in spite of the fact that PCV had reached adult levels [10]. This is in contrast to the situation in adults, where erythropoietin falls when erythropoiesis increases as a result of any kind of therapy for anemia.

Several questions are raised concerning early anemia. Does early anemia give rise to tissue hypoxia? Studies in full-term human babies and rabbits [11] indicate that there is no tissue hypoxia. This may be different in premature infants in whom some studies indicate that they experience tissue hypoxia [12]. The anemia of prematurity may therefore have other causes than the early anemia of full-term healthy babies and young animals.

Early anemia occurs at the time of very rapid growth and, consequently, rapidly expanding blood volume. It has been suggested that anemia is caused by dilution. This would imply that for some reason erythropoiesis could not keep up with the demand. Studies in most mammals contradict this hypothesis. In young pigs [13], mice [14], and rabbits [2, 11, 15] erythropoiesis may proceed at a rate high enough to keep the hemoglobin concentration and PCV volume at adult levels provided they get enough iron. These studies indicate that the cause of early anemia in these species is lack of available iron. It may therefore be concluded that an essential factor in the development of early anemia is lack of availability of essential nutrients. This is further supported by the studies of Rønnholm and Siimes [16] in Helsinki on premature infants. They added human milk protein to human milk and with this fortified human milk preparation they were able to raise the hemoglobin concentration almost 2 g/dl in the supplemented group compared with the control group.

It must also be taken into consideration that during the last part of fetal life and early extrauterine life, there are changes both in sites of erythropoietin production and of hematopoiesis. Erythropoietin production changes from the liver to the kidneys and erythropoiesis from the liver to the bone marrow. These changes occur at different times related to birth in different species. So far, no data definitely prove that a change of erythropoietin production or erythropoiesis site limits the capacity of the erythron.

Effects of Hypertransfusion and Iron Supplementation

In adult mice erythrocyte transfusions depress erythropoiesis almost to zero [17]. Contrary to the adult animal, hypertransfused mice at age 20 days had corrected reticulocyte counts of about 2% and plasma ESF levels significantly above those in hypertransfused adult mice [18]. The plasma erythropoietin levels measured by RIA were, however, the same in adult and neonatal hypertransfused mice, suggesting that nonerythropoietin factors contributed to the increased ESF levels [19].

Iron administration parenterally to nursing young rabbits completely abolished early anemia [2, 11]. Plasma ESF showed, however, a slight continuous rise in the nonanemic rabbits from the 22nd to the 36th days of life [20], indicating that some other factor(s) than anemia stimulate(s) erythropoietin production. Thus, neither high hematocrit levels following hypertransfusion nor normal hematocrit concentrations following iron therapy reduced the ESF activity to zero.

Effects of Hypoxia

Hypoxia given to newborn rabbits increases erythropoietin production [15] but does not increase erythropoiesis or red cell mass (RCM) significantly unless the rabbits were supplied with parenteral iron [2]. In that case RCM/kg increases above what is found in adult rabbits both with and without iron supplementation.

There is no lack of capacity in the erythron to increase erythropoiesis far above what is regularly needed [2]. Also in newborn rats [21] hypoxia increases erythropoietin production after a short period of hypoxia, while neither in the mother nor in the fetuses were the levels increased following chronic hypoxia for 8 days. This suggests that in the fetuses erythropoietin levels after chronic hypoxia are back at the prehypoxic levels too. In newborn mice, erythropoietin increases following short-term hypoxia, but not to the same degree as in adult mice [22].

In the human we have studied the effect of hypoxia by investigating infants with cyanotic heart disease and compared the results with infants with acyanotic heart defects [23]. The studies were performed during diagnostic heart catheterizations. During the first days of life erythropoietin was elevated in most of the babies, both in those with and without cyanosis. In the following 12 weeks, only cyanotic babies had significantly increased erythropoietin levels, but not all of them. One infant, 13 weeks of age, with pulmonary atresia and a PaO_2 rate of 5.9 kPa and a hemoglobin concentration of 22.2 g/dl had serum erythropoietin of 120 mU/ml.

These studies show that full-term infants may also respond to hypoxia with increased erythropoietin production and may also increase erythropoiesis to a degree that maintains hemoglobin concentrations above 20 g/dl.

Erythropoietin or Other Stimulatory Factors in Neonatal Mouse Plasma

Plasma from 20-day-old mice showed a definite increase in Fe^{59} uptake in polycythemic mice [24], a markedly increased ESF activity [25], but also high plasma erythropoietin levels when measured by RIA [19]. The question was raised whether the increased ESF activity could be explained by erythropoietin alone. Nonfractionated plasma from 20-day-old mice and standard erythropoietin showed parallel dose response curves and additive activity in a cell culture assay [26]. In gel filtration the detectable ESF of plasma was eluted in the same position as that of standard erythropoietin. Standard erythropoietin and the ESF of intact plasma and fractionated plasma were identically bound to and eluted from the affinity chromatography column [26]. These studies suggested that erythropoietin alone was responsible for the ESF activity. However, when this plasma was preincubated with antierythropoietin serum, the ESF activity was reduced, but not totally blocked when tested in polycythemic mice or in an in vitro culture, leaving the question open [24].

Insulinlike Growth Factor-1: A Possible Candidate for Nonerythropoietin Activity in Neonatal Plasma

It is well known that erythropoiesis both in vivo and in vitro may be influenced by nonerythropoietin stimulating factors. Since early anemia occurs during a period with rapid growth, it is most likely that factors contributing to growth in general may also influence erythropoiesis. From the studies of Kurtz et al. [27], insulinlike growth factor (IGF-1) may be considered a possible candidate for the nonerythropoietin activity of 20-day-old mouse plasma. Of particular relevance for our studies are the findings that IGF-1 levels are low in fetal and newborn rats, but increase sharply from around the time of weaning [28]. When IGF-1 was given to neonatal rats, the number of colony forming unit-erythroid (CFU_e) in the bone marrow increased, but there was no increase in PCV or reticulocyte counts. The rats also showed increased body weight and skeletal growth [29]. These studies do not prove that IGF-1 is the only candidate for the nonerythropoietin activity of neonatal mouse plasma, but they suggest that IGF-1 may be one of them.

Conclusions

Our studies support the theory that the regulation of erythropoiesis in the neonatal period differs from that observed in the adult. We have documented that early anemia in rabbits is due to lack of available iron. Other workers have found that this is also the case in pigs [13] and mice [14]. Rønnholm and Siimes [16] found that human milk fortified with human milk protein increased hemoglobin concentration in premature infants. Thus nonavailability of essential nutrients is the cause of early anemia in several species and is a contributing factor in the anemia of premature infants. Premature infants have only slightly elevated plasma erythropoietin levels when measured by RIA [6, 7], while the erythropoietic stimulatory activities were significantly elevated when tested with an in vitro culture method [4]. There are still several other possibilities besides lack of erythropoietin which may cause the anemia of prematurity. Exogenous administration of erythropoietin will not necessarily solve that problem. When exposed to short-term hypoxia, the newborn mammal increases its plasma erythropoietin levels. Following chronic hypoxia the levels are not significantly different from controls not exposed to hypoxia. Plasma from 20-day-old mice has high erythropoiesis stimulating activity. This activity is mostly erythropoietin, but nonerythropoietin factors are also operating. IGF-1 is a possible candidate for this nonerythropoietin activity.

References

1. Lucarelli G, Howard D, Stohlman F Jr (1964) Regulation of erythropoiesis. XV. Neonatal erythropoiesis and the effect of nephrectomy J Clin Invest 43: 2195–2203
2. Halvorsen K. Halvorsen S (1973) The "early anemia": its relation to postnatal growth rate, milk feeding, and iron availability. Arch Dis Child 48: 842–849
3. Sanengen T, Holter PH, Hågå A, Hågå P, Meberg A, Halvorsen S, Refsum HE (1987) Perturbation of erythropoiesis during the period of early anemia. A model for studying the regulation of erythropoiesis in the neonatal mammal. In: Rich IN (ed) Molecular and cellular aspects of erythropoietin and erythropoiesis. Springer-Verlag Berlin Heidelberg New York (NATO ASI Series, vol H8)
4. Hågå P, Meberg A, Halvorsen S (1983) Plasma erythropoietin concentrations during the early anemia of prematurity. Acta Paediatr Scand 72: 827–831
5. Hellebostad M, Hågå P and Cotes PM (1988) Serum immunoreactive erythropoietin in healthy normal children. Br J Haematol 70: 247–250
6. Stockman JA III, Greber JE, Clark DA, McClellan K, Garcia JF, Kavey REW (1984) Anemia of prematurity: determinants of the erythropoietin response. J Pediatr 105: 786–792
7. Brown MS, Garcia JF, Phibbs PH, Dallman PR (1984) Decreased response of plasma immunoreactive erythropoietin to "available oxygen" in anemia of prematurity. J Pediatr 105: 793–798
8. Holter PH, Halvorsen S, Refsum HE (1982) Erythrocyte 2,3-DPG, PO_2 50%, and available O_2 during the early post-natal fall in hemoglobin in rabbits. Acta Physiol Scand 116: 7–12
9. Holter PH, Sanengen T, Halvorsen S, Refsum HE (1986) Erythropoiesis-stimulating factor(s), erythropoiesis and erythrocyte 2,3,-diphosphoglycerate in young rabbits with a marked post-natal fall in haemoglobin. Acta Physiol Scand 126: 583–587
10. Meberg A, Hågå P, Johansen M (1980) Plasma erythropoietin levels in mice during the growth period. Br J Haematol 45: 569–574
11. Holter PH, Halvorsen S, Refsum HE (1984) Erythrocyte 2,3-diphosphoglycerate, $PO_2$50%, and available oxygen in young rabbits with and without postnatal fall in hemoglobin. Pediatr Res 18: 154–157
12. Wardrop CAJ, Holland BM, Veale KEA, Jones JG, Gray OP (1978) Nonphysiological anemia of prematurity. Arch Dis Child 53: 855–860

13. Talbot RB, Swenson MJ (1970) Blood volume of pigs from birth through 6 weeks of age. Am J Physiol 218: 1141–1144
14. Jacobson LO, Marks EK, Gaston EO (1959) Studies on erythropoiesis. XII. The effect of transfusion induced polycythemia in the mother on the fetus. Blood 14: 644–653
15. Halvorsen K, Halvorsen S (1974) The regulation of erythropoiesis in the suckling rabbit. Pediatr Res 8: 176–183
16. Rønnholm KAR, Siimes MA (1985) Haemoglobin concentration depends on protein intake in small preterm infants fed human milk. Arch Dis Child 60: 99–104
17. Filmanowics E, Gurney CV (1961) Studies on erythropoiesis. XVI. Response to a single dose of erythropoietin in polycythemiec mice. J Lab Clin Med 57: 65–70
18. Sanengen T, Halvorsen S (1985) Regulation of erythropoiesis during rapid growth. Br J Haematol 61: 273–279
19. Sanengen T, Clemons GK, Halvorsen S, Widness JA (1989) Immunoreactive erythropoietin and erythropoiesis stimulating factor(s) in plasma from hypertransfused neonatal and adult mice. Studies with a radioimmunoassay and a cell culture assay for erythropoietin. Acta Physiol Scand (In press)
20. Sanengen T, Halvorsen S, Refsum HE (1987) Regulation of erythropoiesis in suckling rabbits with and without postnatal anemia: partial suppression of production/release of erythropoiesis stimulating factor(s) by iron supplements. Pediatr Res 21: 1–4
21. Meberg A (1980) Plasma erythropoietin levels in fetal and newborn rats: response to hypoxia. Exp Hematol 8: 615–619
22. Meberg A, Hågå P (1981) Plasma erythropoietin levels in mice. Response to hypoxia at different ages. Scand J Clin Lab Invest 41: 231–235
23. Hågå P, Cotes PM, Till JA, Shinebourne EA, Halvorsen S (1987) Is oxygen supply the only regulator of erythropoietin levels? Serum immunoreactive erythropoietin during the first 4 months of life in term infants with different levels of arterial oxygenation. Acta Pediatr Scand 76: 907–913
24. Sanengen T, Myhre K, Halvorsen S (1987) Erythropoietic factors in plasma from neonatal mice. In vivo studies by the exhypoxic polycythaemic mice assay for erythropoietin. Acta Physiol Scand 129: 381–386
25. Widness JA, Sanengen T, Hågå P, Clemons GK, Myhre K, Halvorsen S (1989) Correlation of plasma erythropoietic stimulatory factor(s) and immunoreactive erythropoietin levels during rapid growth in the mouse. Acta Physiol Scand (In press)
26. Sanengen T, Halvorsen S (1987) Plasma erythropoiesis stimulating factor(s) in neonatal mice: in vitro dose response and chromatography studies. Pediatr Res 21: 148–151
27. Kurtz A, Jelkmann W, Bauer C (1982) A new candidate for the regulation of erythropoiesis. Insulin-like growth factor I. FEBS Lett 149: 105–108
28. Sara VR, Hall K, Menolascino S, Sjøgren B, Wetterberg L, Müntzing K, Oldfors A, Sourander P (1986) The influence of maternal protein deprivation on the developmental pattern of serum immunoreactive insulin-like growth factor 1 (IGF-1) levels. Acta Physiol Scand 126: 391–395
29. Philipps AF, Persson B, Hall K, Lake M, Skottner A, Sanengen T, Sara V (1988) The effects of biosynthetic insulin like growth factor-1 supplementation on somatic growth, maturation and erythropoiesis on the neonatal rat. Pediatr Res 23: 298–305

Pathophysiology of Erythropoiesis

Physiological Studies of Erythropoietin in Plasma

P. M. Cotes

Introduction

Estimates of immunoreactive erythropoietin (EPO) in serum (siEPO) have been used as a tool to explore the physiology of secretion of EPO. This paper summarizes some of our findings in man and relates them to the generally accepted model of the EPO system as a biological feedback loop in which a reduction of tissue oxygen supply activates an as yet unidentified oxygen sensor closely associated with sites of production of EPO, and leads to increased production of the hormone which in turn stimulates the bone marrow to increase the output of new red cells. Thus oxygen delivery is restored to normal. Hyperoxia leads to an increased oxygen supply to the sensor with decreased production of EPO (Fig. 1).

Control of the Concentration of Erythropoietin in Plasma

The amount of EPO in the plasma compartment (Fig. 1) is determined by the balance between its entry and removal. Entry is from sites of formation, mainly in kidney peritubular cells [27] in the adult, with some, perhaps 10%, extrarenal (probably hepatic) production. Whereas the production of EPO is controlled by an oxygen sensor, removal is both by specific effector receptors on committed erythroid progenitors, BFU-E and CFU-E [26] and by non-effector receptors, not necessarily specific for the hormone and perhaps including degradative enzymes. Information about the production and removal of endogenous plasma EPO in man may be derived from studies of the fate of administered EPO (prepared by recombinant DNA technology) [16]. Some EPO, normally 0.5–9 IU/day, is excreted in the urine [2, 3]. It is not clear whether this is from direct secretion of EPO into the renal tubules or renal excretion of the plasma hormone.

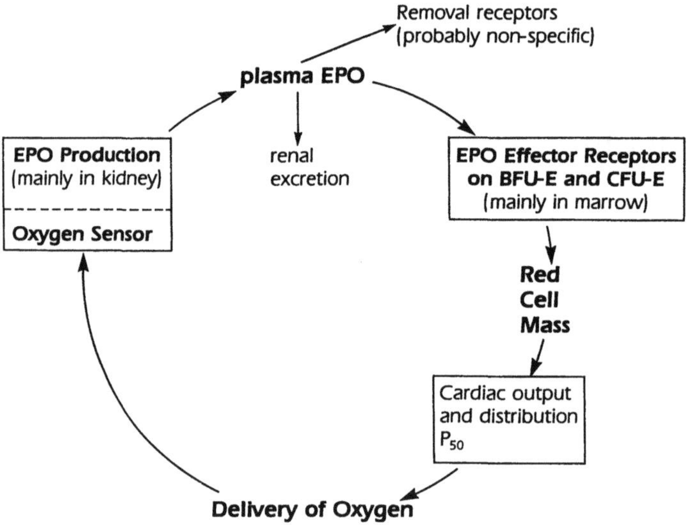

Fig. 1. The erythropoietin system

Estimation of Erythropoietin

The data reviewed in this paper were obtained by radioimmunoassay or by bioassay *in vivo* in exhypoxic polycythaemic mice [8]. The radioimmunoassays were (A) that described by Cotes [6], (B) modification I of method A [13], (C) the assay of Egrie and Lane [18] described in detail as method "a" by Egrie, Cotes, Lane et al. [19] and (D) a modification of method C described by Hågå, Cotes, Till, Minty and Shinebourne [23]. The Second International Reference Preparation of Erythropoietin (IRP) [4] has been used throughout as standard. We found that estimates of EPO in serum are identical whether a sample is fresh or stored at −40°C for up to 1 year. In contrast, whereas estimates in fresh heparinized samples of plasma are identical with those for the corresponding sera, after storage of plasma for 1 year at −40°C, estimates were unreliable and variable with a tendency for EPO in stored plasma samples to give radioimmunoassay dose-dilution lines not parallel to the IRP [10]. For these reasons, our reports of the concentration of EPO in plasma are based on estimates of the hormone in serum.

When any aspect of physiology was explored, we found no differences between the conclusions reached whichever radioimmunoassay method was used. We found similar estimates of EPO for 5 sera each tested on one occasion by methods B and C [19] and small but systematic differences between estimates for 4 sera each tested on 12–16 occasions by methods C and D (Fig. 2). This finding emphasises the experience of endocrinologists that radioimmunoassay estimates are liable to be influenced by change in any component of a radioimmunoassay system.

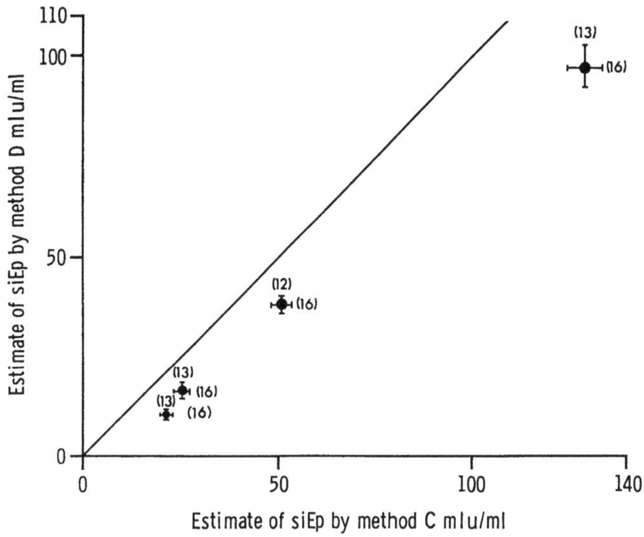

Fig. 2. The relation between geometric mean estimates (with 95 % confidence intervals) of immunoreactive erythropoietin in serum (*siEp*) by methods C and D for four individual serum samples (•) each tested on (*n*) different occasions by method C and on (*n'*) occasions by method D

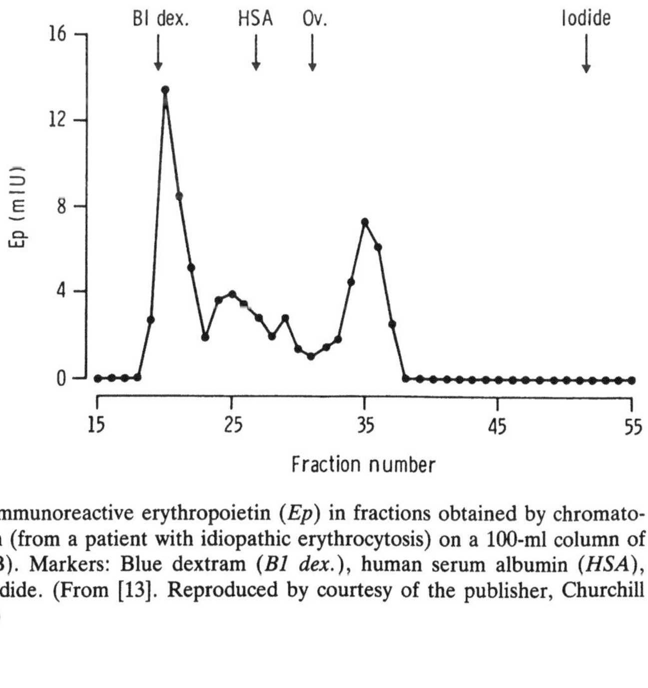

Fig. 3. Distribution of immunoreactive erythropoietin (*Ep*) in fractions obtained by chromatography of 1 ml of serum (from a patient with idiopathic erythrocytosis) on a 100-ml column of Ultrogel ACA 44 (LKB). Markers: Blue dextram (*Bl dex.*), human serum albumin (*HSA*), Ovalbumin (*Ov*) and iodide. (From [13]. Reproduced by courtesy of the publisher, Churchill Livingstone, Edinburgh)

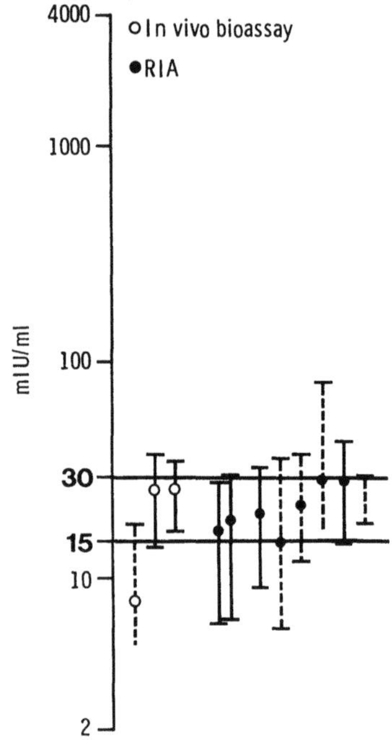

Fig. 4. Recent published estimates of EPO in normal human serum shown as the mean and range (⁝) or calculated 95 % confidence interval ([ ). (Adapted from [7])

Assay validity is considered elsewhere [7] however invalidity occurred unexpectedly for two reasons. These were: damage to ^{125}I radioiodinated tracer EPO in a radioimmunoassay of male mouse submaxillary gland extracts [37, 38] and non-parallelism of dose dilution curves given by a test serum and the IRP [13]. In the first instance, apparently high estimates of EPO were accounted for by tracer damage, and in the second, no estimates could be made but the atypical slope data were subsequently explained by the finding of size heterogeneity in the serum hormone (Fig. 3).

Normal Subjects

Adults

Radioimmunoassay estimates of the concentration of EPO in sera from normal subjects agree well among laboratories which have used assays based on several different antisera, are of the same order as estimates obtained by bioassays *in vivo* and usually fall between 15 and 30 mIU/ml (Fig. 4; for references see [7] and [32]). We found no differences between estimates in men and women, and where such differences have been reported they are small [22]. Nor does the concentration of EPO in serum change with age in adults [30]. During the menstrual cycle, the

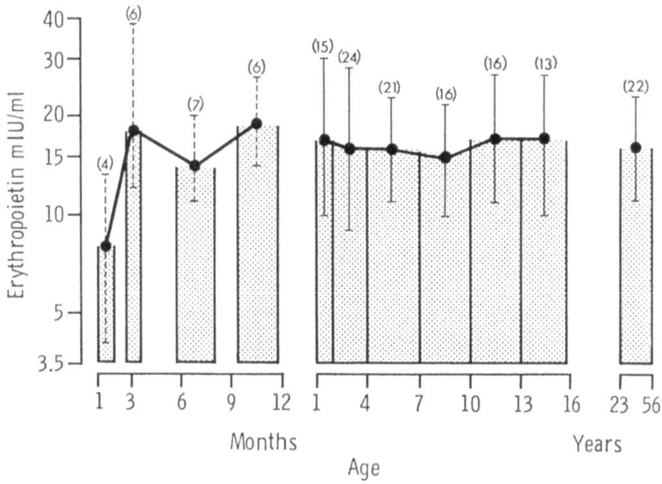

Fig. 5. Estimates of EPO (•) in serum from healthy children and their relation to age. Estimates are shown as arithmetic mean with ranges (⁝) or geometric mean with calculated 95 % range for the observations (I). *Numbers of subjects* are shown in parentheses and *stippled areas* indicate the age range of subjects included in the derivation of each data point. The figure does not include anomalous data for two children in whom siEPO was apparently >256 mIU/ml. (Adapted from [24] and reproduced by courtesy of Blackwell Scientific Publications Ltd., Oxford)

concentrations of EPO in serum samples collected during the follicular and luteal phases are similar [14].

Children

In normal children aged from over 3 months to 16 years [24] estimates of siEPO (Fig. 5) are essentially the same as in adults. These findings were in samples collected from 130 Norwegian children, all of whom were healthy at the time of sampling and differed from the higher values found in samples from only 14 children, age 0.5–1.7 years, attending a "well baby" clinic in Nigeria [41]. However, amongst the Norwegian children there were two outliers. Both were girls age 9–10 years with haemoglobin 15.1 and 13.1 g/dl without evidence of polycythaemia or anaemia, and their siEPO was apparently >256 mIU/ml (Fig. 6). The explanation for this atypical finding will be reported elsewhere. In adults [6] and in children [24] estimates of siEPO are essentially log normally distributed (Fig. 6).

Diurnal Changes

Serum EPO is usually relatively constant (Fig. 7), but a clear pattern of diurnal change was seen in one healthy non-smoking adult male subject (Fig. 8) who was

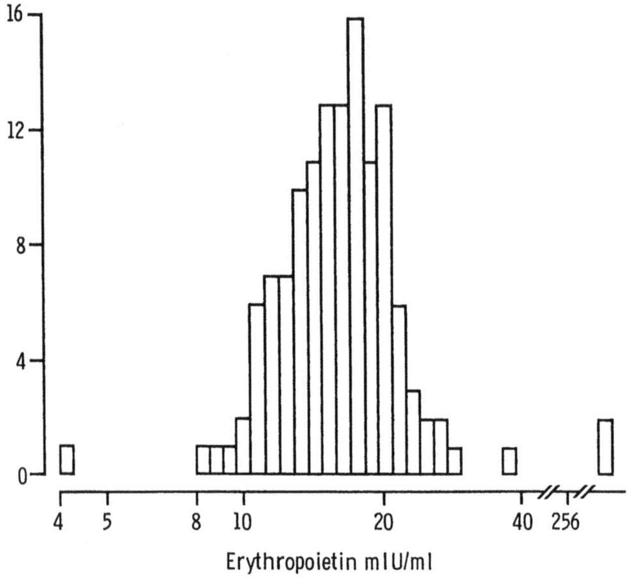

Fig. 6. Histogram showing the distribution of estimates of siEPO on a logarithmic scale for 130 normal children aged 1 month to 16 years. (From [24]. Reproduced by courtesy of Blackwell Scientific Publications Ltd., Oxford)

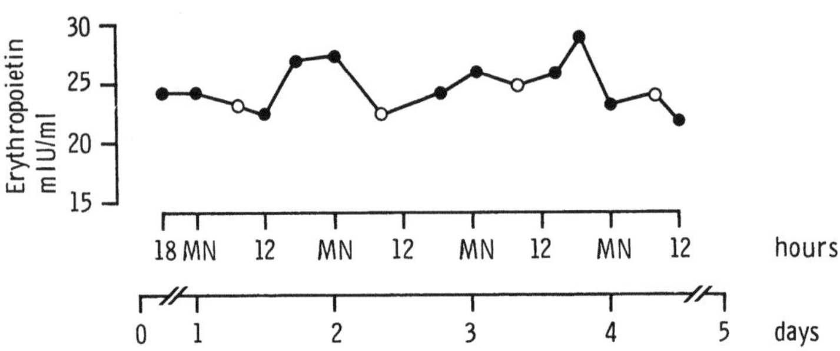

Fig. 7. Estimates of immunoreactive EPO in serum samples collected during a 4-day period from a normal subject when fasting (○) or non-fasting (•). *MN*, midnight. (Adapted from [6] and reproduced by courtesy of Blackwell Scientific Publications Ltd., Oxford)

studied on two occasions [9]. A similar trend was noticed in one other out of a total of eight subjects studied. This phenomenon is probably relatively rare, as it was not seen in another series of 17 normal subjects although it occurred in patients with hypoxic lung disease [30].

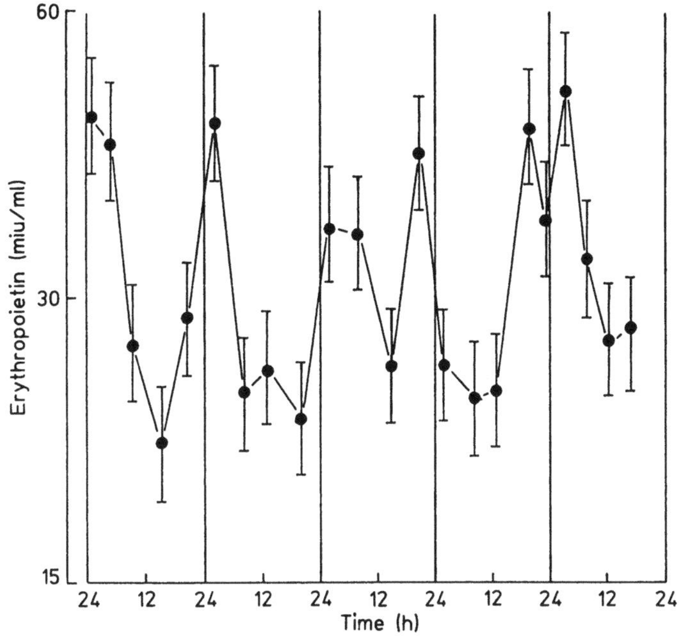

Fig. 8. Diurnal variation in the concentration of immunoreactive EPO in successive 10-ml blood samples from a normal male subject (a non-smoker). Data points show geometric mean estimates from two independent assays (± 1 SE). (From [9]. Reproduced by courtesy of Blackwell Scientific Publications Ltd., Oxford)

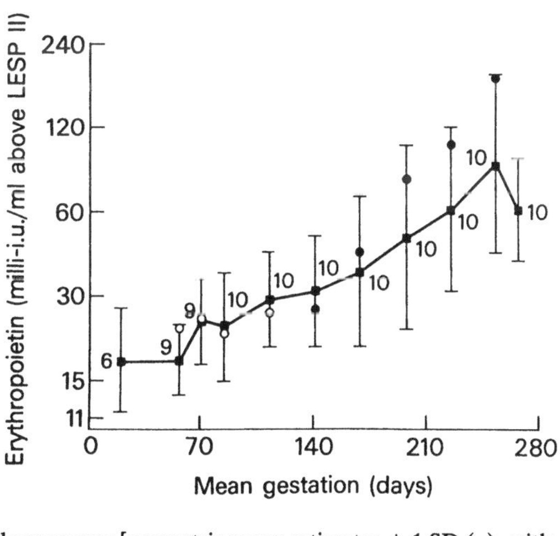

Fig. 9. Estimates of siEPO during normal pregnancy [geometric mean estimates ± 1 SD (■), with number of subjects], and in one subject before (○) and during (●) infusion of salbutamol. The baseline for the assay was a low erythropoietin serum pool (LESPII) [6], later shown to contain 10 mIU EPO/ml [13] (From [14]. Reproduced by courtesy of Blackwell Scientific Publications Ltd., Oxford)

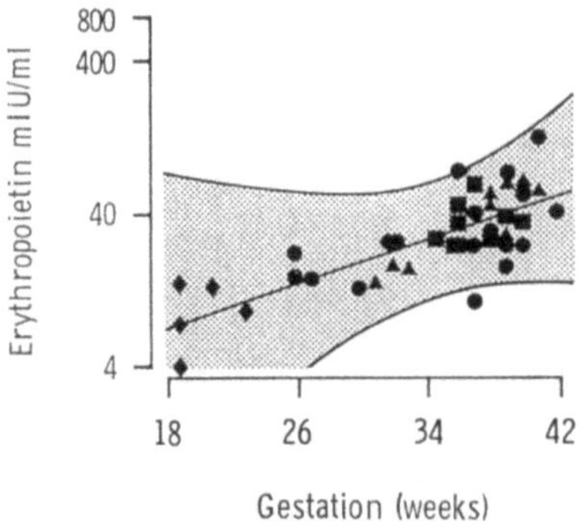

Fig. 10. Estimates of cord siEPO in relation to gestation in normal pregnancy. • Vaginal delivery; ▪ forceps; ▴ Caesarean section; ♦ fetoscopy. The *solid line* shows the predicted value and the *shaded area* represents the 95 % confidence band for single observations of EPO in normal pregnancy. (Adapted from [39] and reproduced by courtesy of Blackwell Scientific Publications Ltd., Oxford)

Pregnancy

In normal pregnancy, siEPO begins to increase some time after 8 weeks and continues to rise with gestation (Fig. 9). Changes are related neither to indicators of haematological and renal function nor to infant birth weight nor to other indicators of endocrine status, with the exception of placental lactogen (HPL). Changes in siEPO and HPL were related ($p<0.00001$) [14].

The β-adrenergic agonist salbutamol induced secretion of EPO in normal rabbits [20, 21]. However, it seemed to have no effect in humans, as in an otherwise normal pregnancy in which this agent was administered to prevent premature labour, both before and during salbutamol infusion estimates of siEPO were similar to estimates in other normal pregnancies (Fig. 9).

The source of the increased plasma EPO in pregnancy is not known. The placenta seems to have been excluded, as there was no consistent decrease in siEPO following removal of the placenta at elective Caesarean section (Cotes, Canning and Lind, unpublished data).

Cord Blood and Amniotic Fluid

In serum from cord blood obtained during gestation (from 19 to 42 weeks) or at delivery in normal pregnancies, the concentration of EPO increased with gestation (Fig. 10) [39]. As early as 24 weeks the fetus responds to severe anaemia with increased siEPO and after correction of the anaemia by transfusion the oxygen feedback control operates and siEPO falls [39]. Estimates of immunoreactive EPO in corresponding maternal and fetal serum samples show no relation between maternal and fetal concentrations (Table 1). Thus in man, as in the sheep [44, 45], placental transfer of EPO does not seem to occur and EPO in amniotic fluid is fetal in origin.

Table 1. Estimates of erythropoietin (EPO) in paired samples of maternal and fetal serum at the time of fetoscopy

Subject	Weeks of gestation	Fetal EPO (mIU/ml)	Maternal EPO (mIU/ml)
1	19	14	18
2	19	4	54
3	19	8	18
4	21	14	27
5	24	10	33
6[a]	24	118*	59
	27	9	63
	30	20	69
7[a]	26	340*	44
	27	53	51
	28	536*	50

From [39]. Reproduced by courtesy of Blackwell Scientific Publications Ltd., Oxford
[a] Nos. 6 and 7 are two fetuses with rhesus haemolytic disease who were transfused in utero
* Above the 95 % level of normal variation for gestational age

Effects of Hypoxic Stimuli in Normal Subjects

Acute Blood Loss

Acute loss of 450 g blood in a normal subject, such as occurs in blood donors, induces an increase in siEPO (Fig. 11, previously unpublished data from Cotes and Brozovic). There was variability among subjects in the magnitude and duration of response, but in some siEPO remained increased 6 days after venesection.

Hypoxia and High Altitude Exposure

In a normal subject exposure to air with oxygen content reduced to 11 % by dilution with nitrogen led to an increase in siEPO perceptible after 2 h (Fig. 12) (previously unpublished data from Cotes and Milledge). We wondered whether the siEPO response would be altered by repeated exposure to hypoxia, and data comparing the effects of exposure to 4500 m on 2 successive days were obtained from samples collected by Dr. J.S. Milledge during an expedition to Pike's Peak, Colorado. Estimates of siEPO after 6 h at altitude 4300 m were essentially the same at first exposure (after ascent by road from 1200 m) and at second exposure on the following day after again spending the night at 1200 m.

On initial exposure to a high altitude there is an increase in siEPO but with continued exposure, by 3 or 4 days, siEPO tends to decrease. This was described by Abbrecht and Littell [1], but inadequate sensitivity of the bioassay prevented estimation of EPO in the baseline or late samples. Milledge and Cotes [29] used a

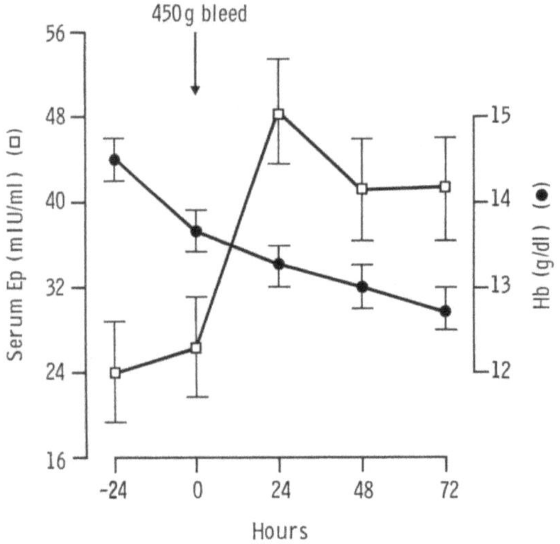

Fig. 11. Changes in serum immunoreactive erythropoietin (*Ep*) and haemoglobin following acute blood loss (450 g) in 16 normal donors. Data points show mean estimates (data of Cotes and Brozovic)

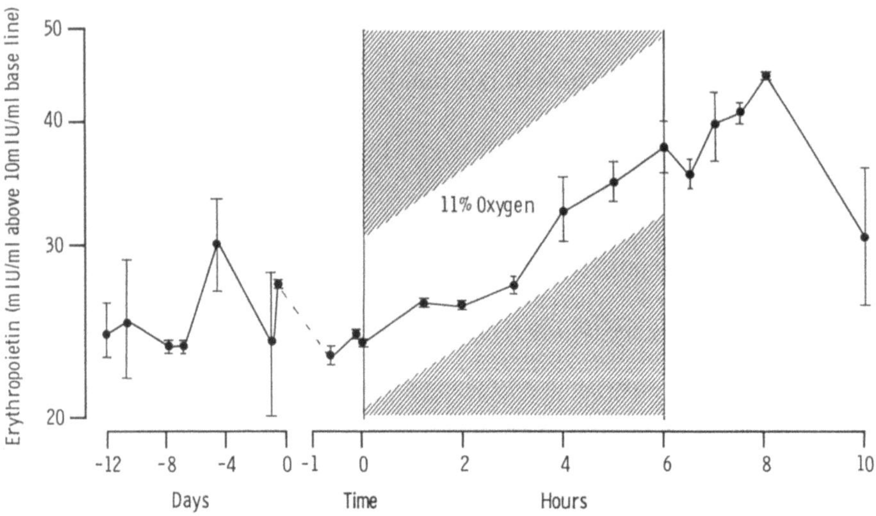

Fig. 12. The effect of breathing 11 % oxygen on siEPO in a normal subject. Estimates are the geometric mean and range from two independent assays (data of Cotes and Milledge)

radioimmunoassay to estimate EPO and confirmed Abbrecht and Littell's findings, and showed that with continuing high altitude exposure siEPO could return to pre-exposure sea level concentrations, although there was almost certainly still incomplete compensation for the hypoxia (Fig. 13). With more severe hypoxia from higher altitude (6300 m for 2–4 weks and some 4–6 weeks at altitude above 4500 m) siEPO remained increased above sea level values [29].

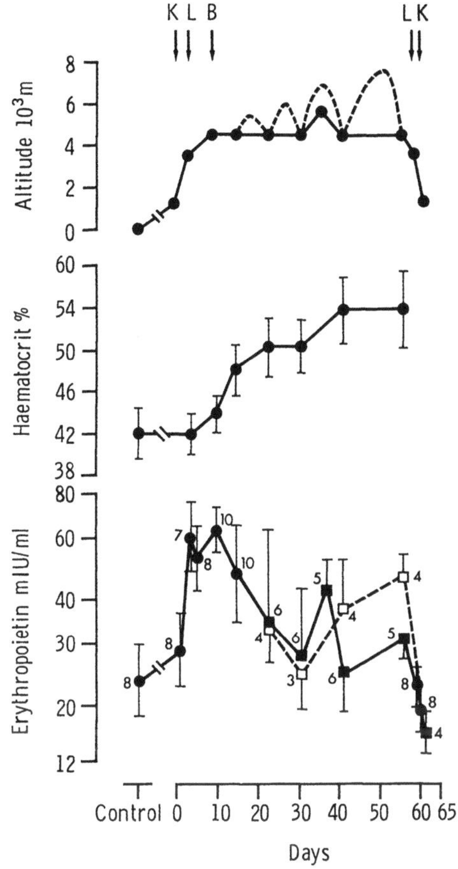

Fig. 13. Mount Kongur expedition. Top: *solid line,* altitude, all subjects; *dotted lines,* additional altitude reached by climbers. Centre: *Filled circles,* mean haematocrit for all subjects ± SD. Bottom: estimates of siEPO as geometric mean and interquartile range for all subjects *(filled circles)*, for climbers *(open squares)*, and for scientists *(filled squares)*. Numbers of subjects are indicated beside each observation. *Arrows* indicate days of travel to Kashgar (*K*), Karakol Lakes (*L*), and base camp (*B*). (From [29]. Reproduced by courtesy of the American Physiological Society)

Anaemias

Anaemias not Associated with Renal Disease

In anaemias (excluding renal disease) siEPO increases with increasing severity of anaemia (Fig. 14). Patients with hypoplastic anaemias tend to have higher concentrations of EPO in plasma than patients with other anaemias. In ten adults with acquired aplastic anaemia (Hb 9.0 ± 1.4 g/dl, mean ± SD), siEPO was 408 mIU/ml (geometric mean) range 180–2700 mIU/ml; and in eight samples from six children with Fanconi's anaemia (Hb 6.9 ± 1.9 g/dl, mean + SD); siEPO was 4.5 IU/ml (geometric mean) range 1.3–17.0 IU/ml.

Amongst conditions in which we found no evidence for impaired formation of EPO are rheumatoid arthritis (Fig. 15), protein energy malnutrition [41], the anaemia induced by experimental infection with human parvovirus (B19) [33], and bronchial cancer, investigated as a model of the anaemias associated with neoplastic disease [35].

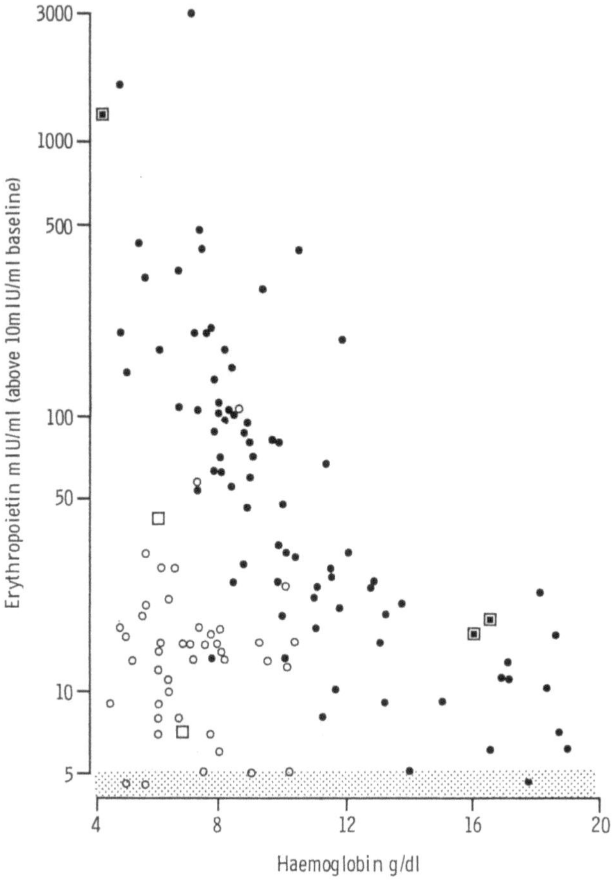

Fig. 14. Haemoglobin and siEPO in patients without renal disease (●), with functioning renal transplant (▣) and with anaemia associated with renal failure managed by dialysis [nephric (○) and anephric (□) subjects]. (Data from [12])

Anaemia associated with Renal Disease

Relation Between Haemoglobin and Erythropoietin. In anaemias associated with renal disease siEPO fails to increase with increasing severity of anaemia (Figs. 14 and 16). This is attributed to damage to the main sites of formation of EPO. EPO is present in plasma of anephric subjects (Fig. 14), but secretion of extrarenal EPO is relatively non-responsive to anaemia, although superimposition of an additional hypoxic stress upon a pre-existing renal anaemia can be associated with an increase in siEPO. Transfusion in an anephric subject is associated with a fall in siEPO, so that despite the relative insensitivity of the extrarenal oxygen sensor in increasing extrarenal production of EPO, the feedback switch-off of EPO secretion is intact.

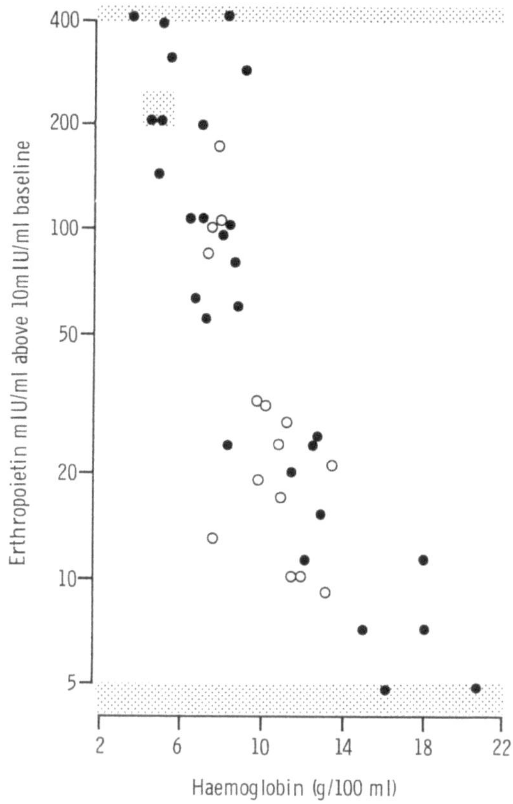

Fig. 15. Haemoglobin and siEPO in patients with rheumatoid arthritis (○) and with other haematological disorders excluding renal failure (•). (Data from [12])

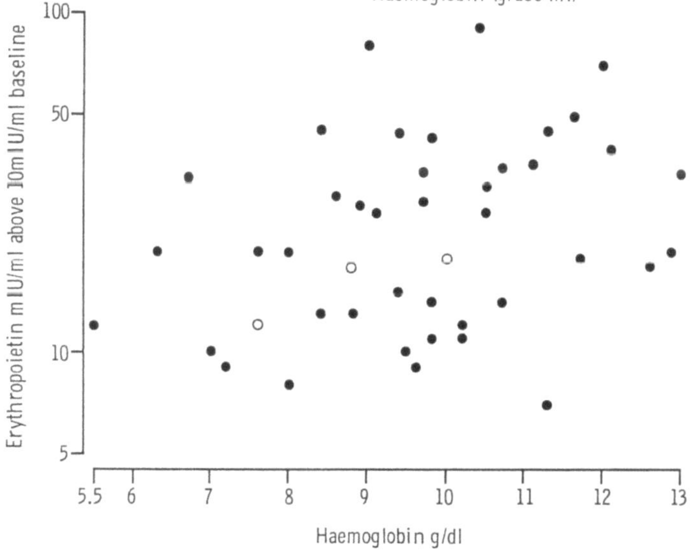

Fig. 16. Serum EPO and haemoglobin in nephric (•) and anephric (○) patients with chronic renal failure maintained by haemodialysis. (Data from [12])

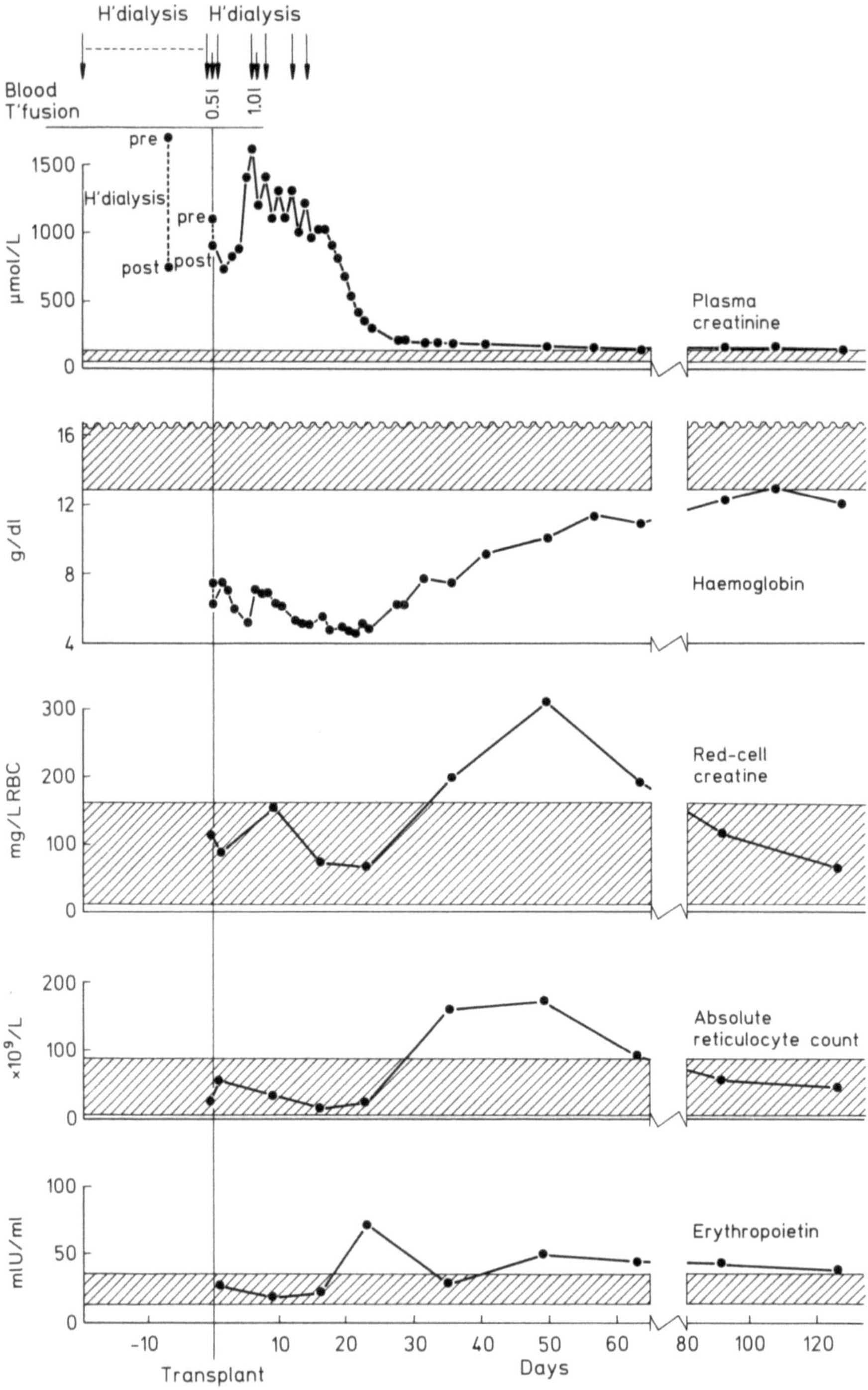
H'dialysis
H'dialysis
Blood
T'fusion
0.5l
1.0l
pre
pre
post
post
H'dialysis
1500
1000
500
0
µmol/L
Plasma
creatinine
16
12
8
4
g/dl
Haemoglobin
300
200
100
0
mg/L RBC
Red-cell
creatine
200
100
0
×10⁹/L
Absolute
reticulocyte count
100
50
0
mIU/ml
Erythropoietin
-10
10
20
30
40
50
60
80
100
120
Transplant
Days

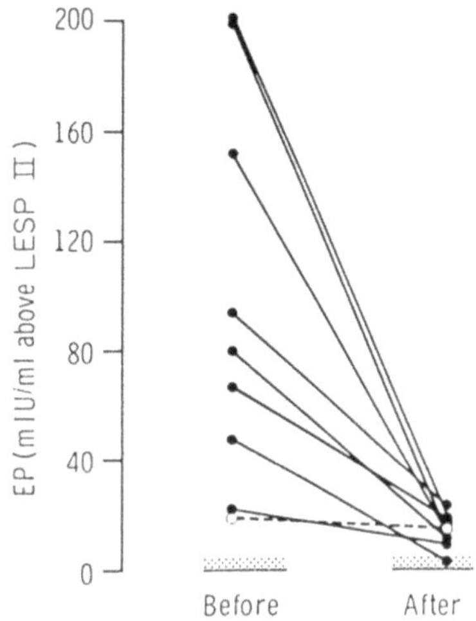

Fig. 18. Serum erythropoietin (*EP*) before and 24-28 h after blood transfusion. In one patient (○) anaemia was associated with renal failure. The baseline for the assay was a low erythropoietin serum pool (LESP II) [6], later shown to contain 10 mIU EPO/ml [13]. (From [6]. Reproduced by courtesy of Blackwell Scientific Publications Ltd., Oxford)

Renal Transplantation

Restoration of renal function by a functioning renal transplant is associated with a return of normal EPO production (Fig. 14). After successful transplantation Rejman et al. [34] noted that reticulocytosis and correction of anaemia were always preceded by an increase in siEPO, presumed to come from the transplanted kidney (Fig. 17).

Correction or Compensation for an Anaemia

Partial correction of an anaemia by transfusion induces a fall in plasma EPO (Fig. 18), as does increasing the partial pressure of oxygen in inspired air in a patient with severe anaemia (Fig. 19). However, it is noteworthy that in anaemia with iron deficiency, administration of iron may induce a fall in plasma EPO before the development of a reticulocyte response and before any correction of the anaemia. This is illustrated (Fig. 20) by the effect of administration of intravenous iron on siEPO in a patient with giant lymph node hyperplasia of the mesentery [5].

Fig. 17. Changes in plasma creatinine, haemoglobin, red cell creatine, reticulocyte count and EPO following successful renal transplant. (From [34]. Reproduced by courtesy of Blackwell Scientific Publications Ltd., Oxford)

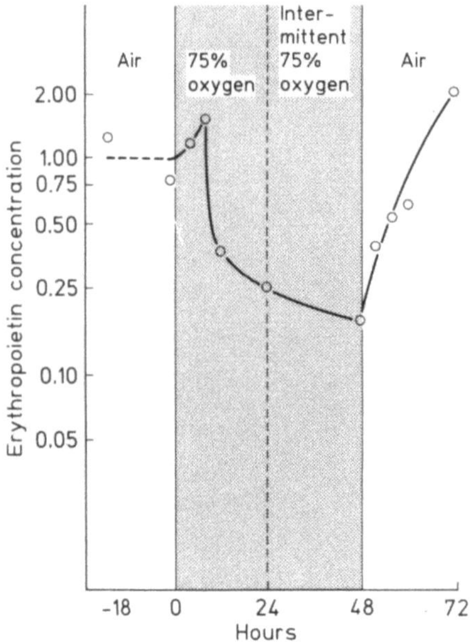

Fig. 19. The effect of increased amounts of oxygen in inspired air on the concentration of EPO in plasma of a patient with paroxysmal nocturnal haemoglobinuria. Estimates of EPO were made by bioassay *in vivo* and in units of research standard A per ml. (From [11])

Polycythaemia

Polycythaemia Vera

In Polycythaemia vera the EPO system functions normally with suppression of EPO production, and mean siEPO is reduced below normal although individual values may be in the range for normal subjects [15] (Fig. 21).

Secondary Polycythaemia

Secondary Polycythaemia with Hypoxia

Two groups of subjects have been studied as models of secondary polycythaemia associated with hypoxia: children with congenital cyanotic heart disease and adults with chronic hypoxic lung disease. Both models show that in chronic hypoxia associated with development of polycythaemia, siEPO is frequently in the normal range, as is also found during prolonged high altitude exposure (page 65 and Fig. 13).

Congenital Cyanotic Heart Disease in Children. In studies carried out in collaboration with Hågå, we found that in 89 % (24 out of 27) of children aged 4 months

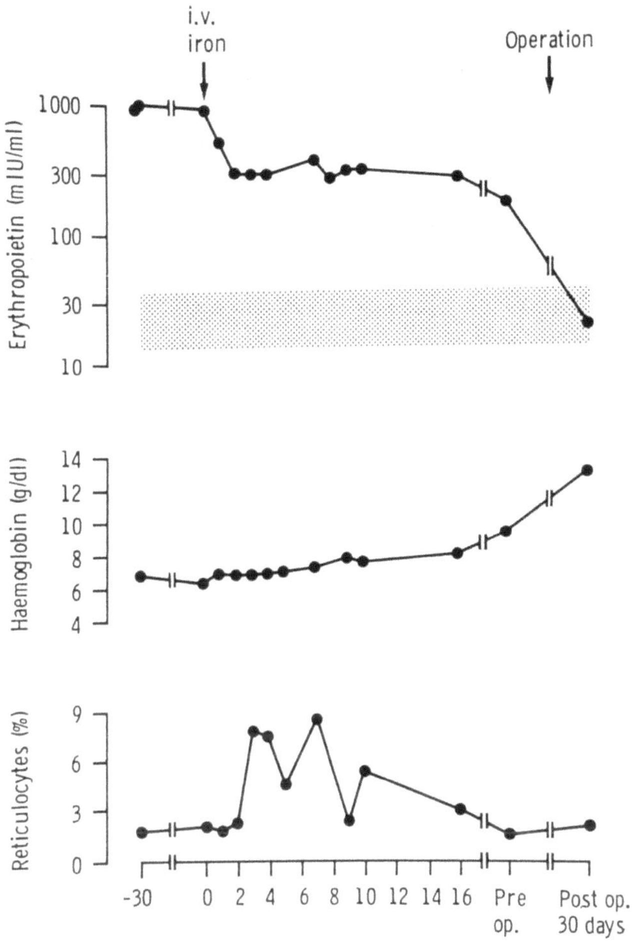

Fig. 20. The effects of intravenous iron and tumour excision on siEPO, haemoglobin and reticulocyte counts in a patient with giant lymph node hyperplasia (Castleman's disease) of the mesentery. (From [5]. Reprinted by courtesy of the American Gastroenterological Association)

to 10 years with congenital cyanotic heart disease, siEPO was the same as in children with acyanotic congenital heart disease and normal adults [23] (Fig. 22). The finding of a normal concentration in the cyanotic group was unexpected, as these children were severely hypoxic with PaO_2 in the range 5.0–8.9 kP_a. Compensatory mechanisms clearly operated in these children, manifest by increases in haemoglobin, haematocrit, P_{50} and arterial oxygen content compared with children with acyanotic congenital heart disease. Nonetheless, Hågå points out that compensation for hypoxia is almost certainly incomplete, as growth is impaired, although not significantly more than in acyanotic children. In the cyanotic children,

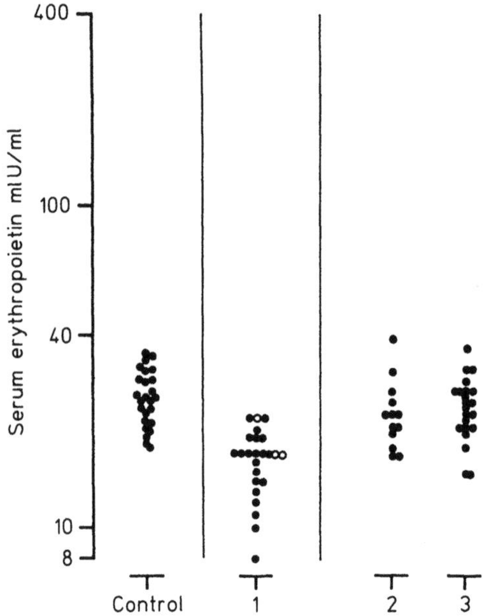

Fig. 21. Serum immunoreactive EPO in patients with polycythaemia vera (*1*) and with relative polycythaemia with raised packed red cell volume, normal red cell mass and low plasma volume (*2*) or normal plasma volume (*3*). Controls were normal subjects. (Data from [15]. Reprinted by permission of the New England Journal of Medicine)

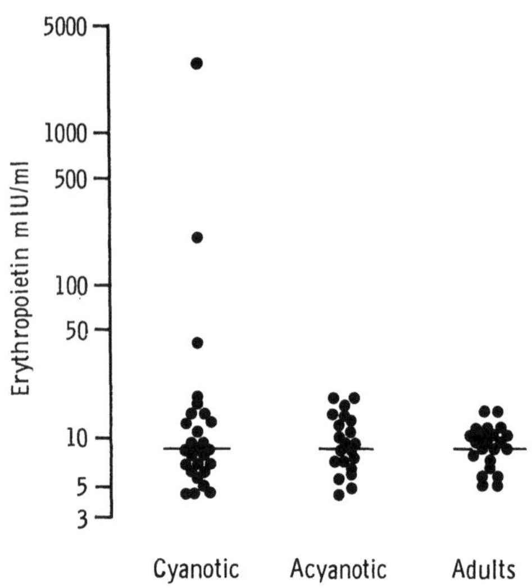

Fig. 22. Serum immunoreactive EPO in cyanotic and acyanotic children with congenital heart disease and in normal adults. *Horizontal lines* show geometric mean estimates (omitting the two highest values in the cyanotic group). (Adapted from [23])

as in the adult exposed to a high altitude, an increase in the severity of hypoxia (as occurs in climbers on ascent to higher altitudes, see Fig. 13) is followed by an increase in siEPO.

Chronic Hypoxic Lung disease. Serum immunoreactive EPO was increased in 69 % of 16 patients with chronic hypoxic lung disease and secondary polycythaemia [40].

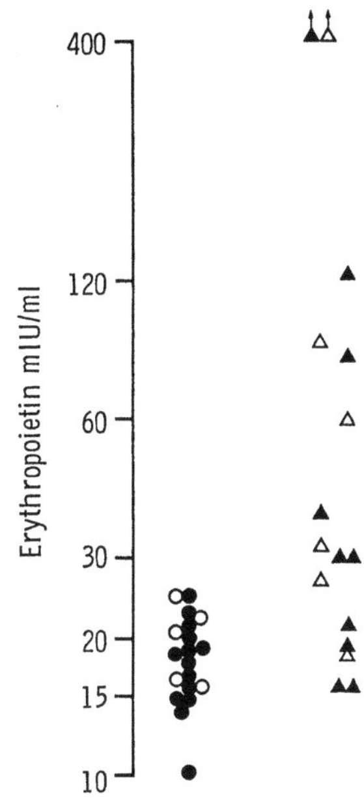

Fig. 23. Estimates of siEPO in samples from normal healthy subjects (● men; ○ women) and from patients with chronic hypoxic lung disease and compensatory polycythaemia (▲ men; △ women)

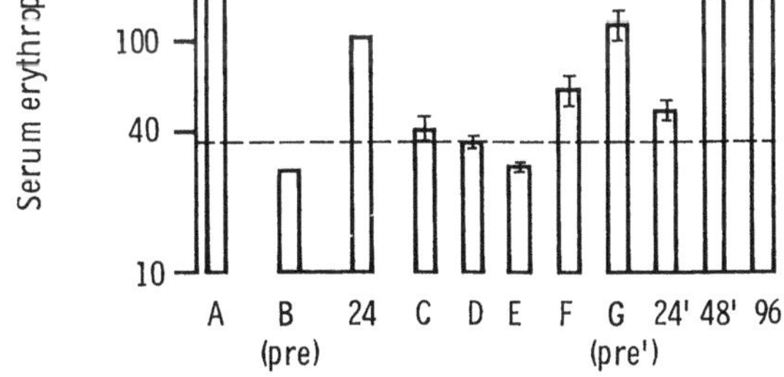

Fig. 24. Estimates of siEPO in a patient with erythrocytosis of unknown cause, showing increased and normal values. Values for siEPO are geometric means and ranges (*bars*); values for *in vivo* biological activity are mean potency and 95 % confidence limits (*bar* and *closed circle*). *A – G*, successive random samples of serum tested; *pre*, level of siEPO immediately before a 450-ml venesection; *24*, number of hours after acute blood loss; *pre', 24', 48', 96'*, as above in a study carried out on a different occasion. The *broken line* indicates the upper 95 % confidence limit of estimates of siEPO levels in normal control subjects. (From [15]. Reprinted by permission of the New England Journal of Medicine)

In the remaining 31 % it was in the normal range (Fig. 23). Amongst these patients we found no means to predict whether siEPO would be increased or normal. But reduction of red cell mass by erythrapheresis was associated with an increase in siEPO, suggesting that polycythaemia may have induced a compensatory decrease in siEPO.

Secondary Polycythaemia with Inappropriate Overproduction of Erythropoietin

Polycythaemia from inappropriate overproduction of EPO from a normal or ectopic site is corrected by removal of a localized lesion producing EPO. In some instances, which may be familial (e.g. [25]), no localized EPO-secreting lesion is found. These cases are diagnosed on the basis of an abnormally increased concentration of EPO in serum, and in one such case the abnormality was intermittent (Fig. 24). This has implications for diagnosis.

Relative Polycythaemia

An increased haematocrit without an increase in total red cell mass (sometimes defined as relative polycythaemia) is associated with normal concentrations of EPO in serum [15] (Fig. 21).

Discussion

The large-scale production of human EPO by recombinant DNA technology has made new reagents available which permit the radioimmunoassay of EPO in unconcentrated body fluids without the need for scarce, highly purified native human EPO from urine [19]. Data from such radioimmunoassays, as well as from assays using reagents from urinary EPO, has increased our understanding of the EPO system and is of value in the investigation and management of polycythaemias of unknown aetiology. The human hormone is essentially recognized as a protein with the structure and biological properties of material which was first isolated from human urine by Miyake et al. [31]. We know less about the characteristics of plasma forms of the hormone. Lukowsky and Painter [28] and Dorado et al. [17] have demonstrated charge heterogeneity in EPO from sheep plasma and human urine, and Cotes et al. [14] and Sherwood et al. [36] found size heterogeneity of immunoreactive EPO in a small number of human serum samples. The heterogeneity of other glycoprotein hormones is well recognized [42, 43] and there is clearly a need for more information about qualitative and quantitative changes in plasma forms of EPO.

Acknowledgements. Nearly all of the work drawn together here was carried out in collaboration with others, whom I thank unreservedly. I also thank Miss C.E. Canning and Mr. R.C. Tam for technical help and the copyright holders for permission to reproduce previously published material.

References

1. Abbrecht PH, Littell JK (1972) Plasma erythropoietin in men and mice during acclimatization to different altitudes. J Appl Physiol 32: 54–58
2. Adamson JW, Alexanian R, Martinez C, Finch CA (1966) Erythropoietin excretion in normal man. Blood 28: 354–364
3. Alexanian R (1966) Urinary excretion of erythropoietin in normal men and women. Blood 28: 344–353
4. Annable LM, Cotes PM, Mussett MV (1972) The second international reference preparation of erythropoietin, human urinary, for bioassay. Bull WHO 47: 99–112
5. Bjarnason I, Cotes PM, Knowles S, Reid C, Wilkins R, Peters TJ (1984) Giant lymph node hyperplasia (Castleman's disease) of the mesentery. Observations on the associated anemia. Gastroenterology 87: 216–223
6. Cotes PM (1982) Immunoreactive erythropoietin in serum. I. Evidence for the validity of the assay method and the physiological relevance of estimates. Br J Haematol 50: 427–438
7. Cotes PM (1987) The estimation of erythropoietin (Epo): principles, problems and progress. In: Rich IN (ed) Molecular and cellular aspects of erythropoietin and erythropoiesis. NATO ASI Series, vol H8, Springer, Berlin Heidelberg New York, pp 377–387
8. Cotes PM, Bangham DR (1961) Bioassay of erythropoietin in mice made polycythaemic by exposure to air at a reduced pressure. Nature 191: 1065–1067
9. Cotes PM, Brozovic B (1982) Diurnal variation of serum immunoreactive erythropoietin in a normal subject. Clin Endocrinol 17: 419–422
10. Cotes PM, Canning CE (1982) Stability of immunoreactive erythropoietin in blood, plasma and serum. Blood 60 (Suppl 1]: 85a
11. Cotes PM, Lowe RD (1963) The influence of renal ischaemia on red-cell formation. Mem Soc Endocrinol 13: 187–194
12. Cotes PM, Brozovic B, Mansell M, Samson DM (1980) Radioimmunoassay of erythropoietin in human serum: Validation and application of an assay system. Experimental Hematology 8: Suppl. 8, 292
13. Cotes PM, Canning CE, Gaines Das RE (1983) Modification of a radioimmunoassay for human serum erythropoietin to provide increased sensitivity and investigate nonspecific serum responses. In: Hunter WM, Corrie JET (eds) Immunoassays for clinical chemistry. Churchill Livingstone, Edinburgh, pp 106–112, 124–127
14. Cotes PM, Canning CE, Lind T (1983) Changes in serum immunoreactive erythropoietin during the menstrual cycle and normal pregnancy. Br J Obstet Gynaecol 90: 304–311
15. Cotes PM, Dore CJ, Yin JAL, Lewis SM, Messinezy M, Pearson TC, Reid C (1986) Determination of serum immunoreactive erythropoietin in the investigation of erythrocytosis. N Engl J Med 315: 283–287
16. Cotes PM, Pippard MJ, Reid CDL, Winearls CG, Oliver DO, Royston JP (1989) Characterization of the anaemia of chronic renal failure and the mode of its correction by erythropoietin (r-HuEPO). An investigation of the pharmacokinetics of intravenous r-HuEPO and its effects on erythrokinetics. Q J Med New Series 70: 113–137
17. Dorado M, Langton AA, Brandan NC, Espada J (1972) Electrophoretic behavior of erythropoietin in polyacrylamide gel. Biochem Med 6: 238–245

18. Egrie JC, Lane J (1987) Development of a radioimmunoassay for erythropoietin using recombinant erythropietin-derived reagents. In: Rich IN (ed) Molecular and cellular aspects of erythropoietin and erythropoiesis. NATO ASI Series, vol H8. Springer, Berlin Heidelberg New York pp 395–407
19. Egrie JC, Cotes PM, Lane J, Gaines Das RE, Tam RC (1987) Development of radioimmunoassays for human erythropoietin using recombinant erythropoietin as tracer and immunogen. J Immunol Methods 99: 235–241
20. Fink GD, Fisher JW (1977) Stimulation of erythropoiesis by beta adrenergic agonists. I. Characterization of activity in polycythemic mice. J Pharmacol Exp Ther 202: 192–198
21. Fink GD, Fisher JW (1977) Stimulation of erythropoiesis by beta adrenergic agonists. II. Mechanism of action. J Pharmacol Exp Ther 202: 199–208
22. Garcia JF, Ebbe SN, Hollander L, Cutting HO, Miller ME, Cronkite EP (1982) Radioimmunoassay of erythropoietin: circulating levels in normal and polycythemic human beings. J Lab Clin Med 99: 624–635
23. Hågå P, Cotes PM, Till JA, Minty BD, Shinebourne EA (1987) Serum immunoreactive erythropoietin in children with cyanotic and acyanotic congenital heart disease. Blood 70: 822–826
24. Hellebostad M, Hågå P, Cotes PM (1988) Serum erythropoietin in healthy normal children. Br J Haematol 70: 247–250
25. Hellman A, Rotoli B, Cotes PM, Luzzatto L (1983) Familial erythrocytosis with overproduction of erythropoietin. Clin Lab Haematol 5: 335–342
26. Sawada K, Krantz SB, Sawyer ST, Civin CI (1988) Quantitation of specific binding of erythropoietin to human erythroid colony-forming cells. J Cell Physiol 137: 337–345
27. Lacombe C, Da Silva J-L, Bruneval P, Camilleri J-P, Bariety J, Tambourin P, Varet B (1988) Identification of tissues and cells producing erythropoietin in the anemic mouse. Contr Nephrol 66: 17–24
28. Lukowsky WA, Painter RH (1972) Studies on the role of sialic acid in the physical and biological properties of erythropoietin. Can J Biochem 50: 909–917
29. Milledge JS, Cotes PM (1985) Serum erythropoietin in humans at high altitude and its relation to plasma renin. J Appl Physiol 59: 360–364
30. Miller ME, Garcia JF, Cohen RA, Cronkite EP, Moisia G, Acevedo J (1981) Diurnal levels of immunoreactive erythropoietin in normal subjects and subjects with chronic lung disease. Br J Haematol 49: 189–200
31. Miyake T, Kung CK-H, Goldwasser E (1977) Purification of human erythropoietin. J Biol Chem 252: 5558–5564
32. Mizoguchi H, Otha K, Suzuki T, Murakami A, Ueda M, Saski R, Chiba H (1987) Basic conditions for radioimmunoassay of erythropoietin and plasma levels of erythropoietin in normal subjects and anemic patients. Acta Haematol Jpn 50: 15–24
33. Potter CG, Potter AC, Hatton CSR, Chapel HM, Anderson MJ, Pattison JR, Tyrrel DAJ, Higgins PG, Willman JS, Parry HF, Cotes PM (1987) Variation of erythroid and myeloid precursors in the marrow and peripheral blood of volunteer subjects infected with human parvovirus (B19). J Clin Invest 79: 1486–1492
34. Rejman ASM, Grimes AJ, Cotes PM, Mansell MA, Joekes AM (1985) Correction of anaemia following renal tranplantation: serial changes in serum immunoreactive erythropoietin, absolute reticulocyte count and red-cell creatine levels. Br J Haematol 61: 421–431
35. Schreuder WO, Ting WC, Smith S, Jacobs A (1984) Testosterone, erythropoietin and anaemia in patients with disseminated bronchial cancer. Br J Haematol 57: 521–526
36. Sherwood JB, Carmichael LD, Goldwasser E (1988) The heterogeneity of circulating human erythropoietin. Endocrinology 122: 1472–1477
37. Tam RC, Bedwell J, Reed P, Cotes PM (1988) Anomalous radioimmunoassay estimates of submaxillary gland erythropoietin. Biochem Soc Trans 16: 564–565
38. Tam RC, Bedwell J, Cotes PM, Reed PJ (1989) Sexual dimorphism of erythropoietin degrading activity in mouse salivary gland extracts. Exp Hematol 17: 160–163

39. Thomas RM, Canning CE, Cotes PM, Linch DC, Rodeck CH, Rossiter CE, Huehns ER (1983) Erythropoietin and cord blood haemoglobin in the regulation of human fetal erythropoiesis. Br J Obstet Gynaecol 90: 795–800
40. Wedzicha JA, Cotes PM, Empey DW, Newland AC, Royston JP, Tam RC (1985) Serum immunoreactive erythropoietin in hypoxic lung disease with and without polycythaemia. Clin Sci 69: 413–422
41. Wickramasinghe SN, Cotes PM, Gill DS, Tam RC, Grange A, Akinyanju OO (1985) Serum immunoreactive erythropoietin and erythropoiesis in protein energy malnutrition. Br J Haematol 60: 515-524
42. Wide L (1985) Median charge and charge heterogeneity of human pituitary FSH, LH and TSH I. Zone electrophoresis in agarose suspension. Acta Endocrinol (Copenh) 109: 181–189
43. Wide L, Hobson B (1987) Some qualitative differences of HCG in serum from early and late pregnancies and trophoblastic diseases. Acta Endocrinol (Copenh) 116: 465–472
44. Zanjani ED, Gordon AS (1971) Erythropoietin production and utilization in fetal goats and sheep. Isr J Med Sci 7: 850–856
45. Zanjani ED, Peterson EN, Gordon AS, Wasserman RR (1974) Erythropoietin production in the fetus: role of the kidney and maternal anaemia. J Lab Clin Med 83: 281–287

Erythropoietin Production in Malignancy

H. JOHANNSEN, A. J. GROSS, and W. JELKMANN

Introduction

The glycoprotein hormone erythropoietin stimulates the proliferation and differentiation of erythrocytic progenitors in bone marrow. Erythropoiesis counterbalances the permanent loss of aged red blood cells. The red cell mass, hemoglobin concentration, and oxygen transport capacity of the blood are relatively constant under physiological conditions. The production of erythropoietin is augmented following phlebotomy, until the mass of red blood cells is restored.

Abnormal erythropoiesis is a frequent complication in malignant diseases. Most of the patients develop anemia. In this chapter some of the mechanisms will be reported which have been implicated previously in the pathogenesis of the anemia associated with malignancy. Of interest are findings from our own laboratory which indicate that serum erythropoietin levels may be abnormally high in acute leukemia. Finally, certain types of tumors are of note in association with secondary polycythemia due to paraneoplastic erythropoietin production.

Anemia Associated with Cancer

Anemia is a frequent complication of cancer even when myelophthisis is absent [9]. Several mechanisms have been implicated in the pathogenesis of this anemia. These include bleeding, hemolysis, a reduced bone marrow response to erythropoietin, and relatively low plasma erythropoietin levels for the degree of anemia [70, 72]. The anemia can be aggravated by the inhibition of erythropoiesis due to the application of cytostatic drugs or by the loss of blood during surgical procedures.

Bone Marrow Erythropoiesis

The failure of the bone marrow to increase red cell production sufficiently is thought to be the most important factor in the pathogenesis of anemia in malignancy. Abnormalities in iron turnover may be partly involved in the inability of the bone marrow to respond [7, 11]. However, impaired release of iron from reticuloendothelial cells resulting in hypoferremia and inappropriate iron supply to the erythron do not fully explain the anemia of chronic diseases [40, 72]. Zucker et al. [72] have observed a reduced in vitro heme-synthesizing capacity of bone marrow suspension cultures from cancer patients, when compared with cultures from either normal individuals or patients with chronic infection or inflammation. More recently, however, Dainiak et al. [9] failed to confirm such primary marrow defect, as both primitive (BFU-E) and more differentiated (CFU–E) erythrocytic progenitors of cancer patients proliferated normally in response to erythropoietin in vitro. Abnormalities were detected neither in the size nor in the degree of hemoglobinization of erythrocytic colonies grown from marrow of cancer patients [9]. However, the possibility cannot be excluded from these in vitro studies that tumor products inhibit the in vivo proliferation of erythrocytic progenitors. Recently, the existence of macrophage-derived factors that suppress the growth of erythrocytic progenitors has been considered in the mechanism underlying the hypoproliferative anemia of chronic diseases [55, 56].

Plasma Erythropoietin Level

The importance of depressed erythropoietin production in the pathogenesis of anemia in malignancy has remained a controversial subject. Some investigators noted no correlation between the level of serum erythropoietin and the degree of anemia in patients with malignancy [15, 70]. Dainiak et al. [9] failed to detect erythropoietin bioactivity in the sera of five severely anemic tumor patients. In contrast with Schreuder et al. [57], Cox et al. [8] have considered reduced erythropoietin levels as the cause of anemia in patients with bronchial cancer. It has been proposed that the increased catabolism and the general impairment of protein synthesis associated with malignant diseases contribute to the depression of the production of erythropoietin [40]. On the other hand, Zucker et al. [72] earlier found a clear correlation between the plasma erythropoietin level and the degree of anemia in most of their patients suffering from malignancies. In addition, there was no difference between the erythropoietin level in malignancy and that in the anemia of iron or folate deficiency. Douglas and Adamson [11] have reported a similar increase in plasma erythropoietin relative to the degree of anemia in patients with malignancy and those with inflammation, although in both groups of patients some of the erythropoietin values were considerably low. Schreuder et al. [57] were the first who measured erythropoietin by radioimmunoassay in malignancy. The serum erythropoietin concentration in patients with broncial cancer was not reduced compared to that in anemic individuals without malignant disease (Fig. 1). Instead, there seemed to be an association of anemia with lowered serum concentrations of testosterone [57].

Most of the earlier results were obtained using bioassays for erythropoietin. Plasma samples may contain toxins and drugs which interfere with the biologic

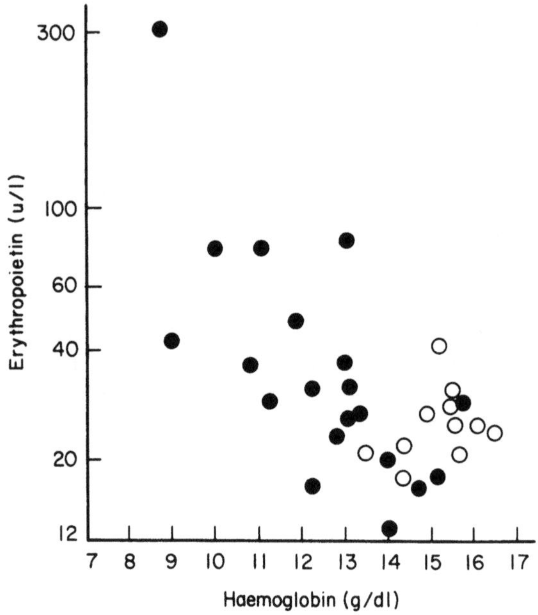

Fig. 1. Semilogarithmic presentation of the serum erythropoietin concentration (radioimmunoassay) as a function of the blood hemoglobin concentration in 20 male patients with bronchial cancer (●) and 11 control subjects (○). (Reproduced from [57])

action of erythropoietin (for references, see [32]). Previous tests were negative for the presence of serum inhibitors of erythropoietin in tumor-bearing patients [70, 72] and mice [10]. In addition, it is evidently of little value to perform a quantitative analysis of the relation between plasma erythropoietin values and blood hemoglobin concentration as long as there is a lack of information on the "normal" erythropoietin concentration in humans suffering from chronic anemia, i.e. in individuals without renal disease, malignancy, infection, inflammation or primary hemopoietic disorder.

Erythropoietin Levels in Leukemia

In leukemia the hemopoietic tissue is the site of neoplastic growth. In the acute forms abnormally high numbers of immature hemopoietic cells are found in the blood. In the chronic forms the numbers of mature white blood cells are increased. In both forms leukemic cells progressively infiltrate the bone marrow. A decrease in the numbers of the erythrocytic progenitors, CFU-E and BFU-E, is usually found in progressive acute myelogenous leukemia (AML) [42]. Yet the anemia in leukemic patients is not always due to the replacement of normal erythrocytic progenitors by leukemic cells [13]. Both the granulocytic and the erythrocytic progenitor compartments are enlarged in the bone marrow of patients suffering from chronic myelogenous leukemia (CML) [13, 21]. The relative number of

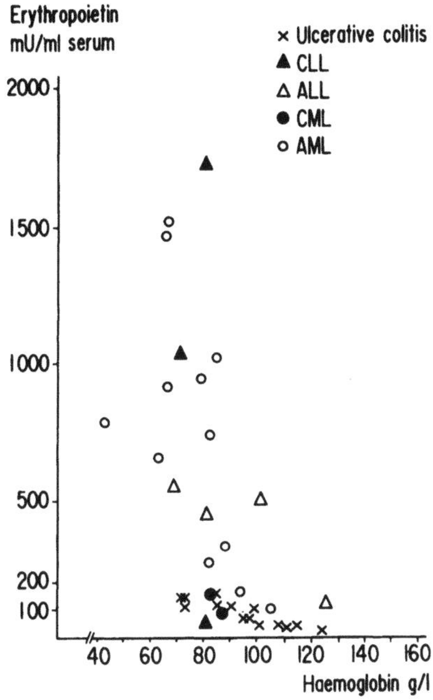

Fig. 2. Serum erythropoietin bioactivity (assay in exhypoxic polycythemic mice) as a function of the blood hemoglobin concentration in anemic patients suffering from ulcerative colitis (14 cases) or leukemia (no. of cases: 3 CLL, 4 ALL, 2 CML, 12 AML). Data are from [33]

marrow CFU-E has been shown to be normal [17] or even elevated [12] in CML. Leukemic cell clones may suppress the differentiation of erythrocytic progenitors [29]. Erythropoietin–independent growth or increased sensitivity to erythropoietin of erythrocytic progenitors was observed in some cases of AML, CML and myeloproliferative disorders but the understanding of these findings is still incomplete [12, 13, 38].

Several investigators have demonstrated increased plasma erythropoietin levels in anemic patients with acute leukemia [54, 64]. Hence, Pavlovic-Kentera et al. [54] concluded that the anemia in leukemia is not primarily due to erythropoietin deficiency.

We have recently studied the level of serum erythropoietin in patients with different types of leukemia [33]. Several of the leukemic patients had considerably higher serum erythropoietin values than similarly anemic patients suffering from chronic bleeding, i.e. patients with ulcerative colitis (Fig. 2). Erythropoiesis is not primarily impaired in ulcerative colitis, although eventually iron deficiency may develop. In contrast with the situation in ulcerative colitis, there was no clear correlation between the serum erythropoietin concentration and the hemoglobin concentration in the group of leukemic patients as a whole. Our observation of relatively low erythropoietin values in anemic patients with CML (Fig. 2) confirms earlier findings by Murphy and Mirand [46] and Fukushima et al. [17]. Hoffman and Zanjani [28] demonstrated in a case of juvenile CML that erythropoiesis remained dependent on erythropoietin. In their study serum erythropoietin decreased when the hemoglobin concentration in blood was normalized. Likewise,

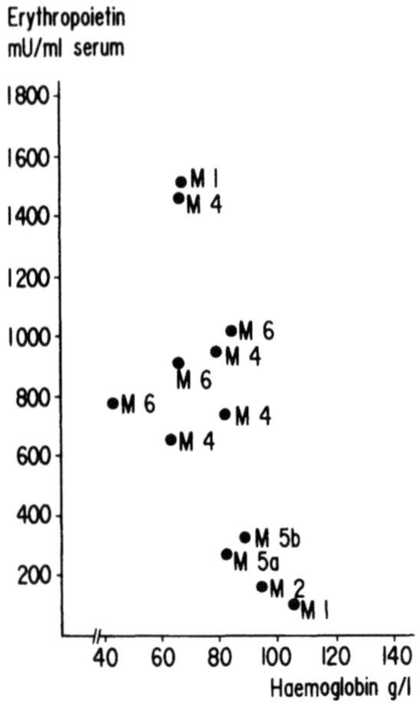

Fig. 3. Serum erythropoietin bioactivity (assay in exhypoxic polycythemic mice) as a function of the blood hemoglobin concentration in AML patients specified according to the FAB classification (AML M1–AML M6). Data are from [33]

the mechanisms normally controlling the production of erythropoietin on the basis of oxygen supply to the tissues still act in acute lymphoblastic leukemia (ALL). In the study by Toogood et al. [66] two of five anemic children with ALL had elevated serum erythropoietin which disappeared after hypertransfusion.

Figure 3 shows the concentration of erythropoietin as a function of the hemoglobin concentration in the blood of AML patients classified according to the French-American-British group [3]. Patients with myelomonocytic leukemia (AML M4) and erythroleukemia (AML M6) had relatively high serum erythropoietin levels. Transfusion with packed red blood cells was earlier found to elicit a significant decrease in serum erythropoietin in a patient with erythroleukemia [18]. Hankins et al. [26] screened 70 murine erythroleukemia cell lines for in vitro production of erythropoietin. Four cell lines from Friend virus-infected mice gave a positive response. Previous attempts have failed to demonstrate erythropoietin production by human erythroleukemia cell lines.

Erythropoietin Production by Neoplasms

Various benign and malignant tumors have been associated with erythrocytosis secondary to the production of erythropoietin by the neoplasms. The incidence of this paraneoplastic syndrome is probably not exactly known, because the action of erythropoietin may be inhibited by the factors involved in the pathomechanism of the anemia of malignancy. Paraneoplastic erythrocytosis can be differentiated from polycythemia vera by the higher plasma erythropoietin concentration, the lack of elevated granulocyte and platelet counts, and the absence of splenomegaly. On the other hand, secondary polycythemia caused by tissue hypoxia is associated with lowered arterial oxygen tension, increased oxygen affinity of the blood or reduced renal blood flow.

Renal Tumors

The kidney is not only the main physiological site of the production of erythropoietin. Erythrocytosis in association with renal tumors has been repeatedly reported [1, 25, 35, 45, 46, 62, 65, 69]. Hammond and Winnick [25] reviewed 340 cases of paraneoplastic erythrocytosis. Thirty-five percent of the patients suffered from renal carcinoma. In a study of 57 patients with renal carcinoma, 63% had elevated plasma erythropoietin levels [62]. The erythropoietin level did neither correlate with tumor grade or stage nor with hematocrit or blood hemoglobin concentration. In the study by Thorling [65] 19 of 25 patients with renal carcinoma and erythrocytosis had increased erythropoietin activity in serum, urine or tumor extract. It is noteworthy, after all, that polycythemia develops only in about 3% of all patients with renal carcinoma [35, 69], and certainly anemia is found more often in this disease.

Recent in vitro hybridization studies have localized erythropoietin mRNA in renal carcinoma cells [5]. The results indicate that the neoplastic cells producing erythropoietin are distinct from the peritubular capillary cells that form erythropoietin mRNA in hypoxia [39, 44].

It has been established that renal carcinoma cells produce erythropoietin directly, and not indirectly by inducing kidney hypoxia. Kvarstein et al. [41] reported a case of erythrocytosis in which the hematocrit and hemoglobin returned to normal after the tumor-bearing kidney was removed. A few months later, erythropoietin increased in the plasma and erythrocytosis developed a new in association with a tumor recurrence. Erythrocytosis and enhanced plasma concentrations of erythropoietin also developed in nude mice receiving lung metastatic transplants from a patient with renal carcinoma [67]. In addition, clear cell and granular cell renal carcinomas grown in culture produce erythropoietin [24, 34, 52, 60, 63].

Blood levels of erythropoietin are elevated in 60%–70% of all patients with Wilms' tumor [36, 47, 48]. Nevertheless, secondary polycythemia is very rarely seen [48, 61]. Erythropoietin bioactivity was demonstrated in Wilms' tumor extracts [58, 61]. Plasma erythropoietin subsides postoperatively unless metastatic foci develop [48]. Thus, measurements of plasma erythropoietin are of diagnostic value in Wilms' tumor patients.

Benign renal tumors have been associated with synthesis of erythropoietin and erythrocytosis [19, 25, 46, 59]. Nephrectomy in such cases usually corrects the hematological abnormality. The mechanism of the stimulation of the production of erythropoietin in renal adenomas and cysts is not known. Perhaps pressure-induced ischemia and hypoxia of the kidney tissue is involved.

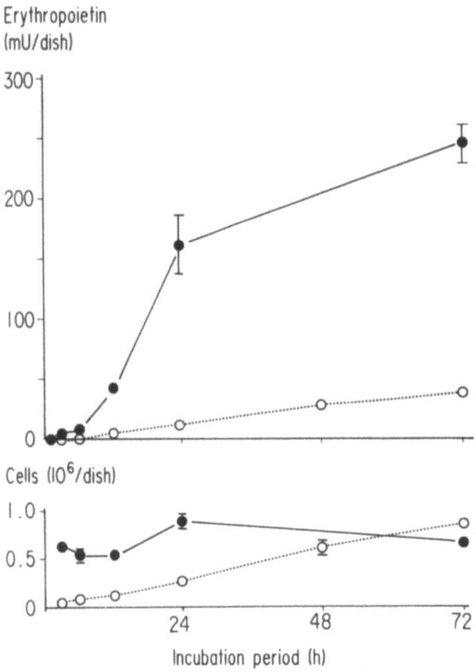

Fig. 4. Accumulation of erythropoietin (radioimmunoassay) in the culture media of confluent (*filled circles*) and proliferating (*open circles*) monolayers of the human hepatoma cell line HepG2 (*upper panel*). The number of cells per dish is given as an index of the density of the cell layer (*lower panel*). The cultures were incubated in 1 ml medium RPMI 1640 supplemented with 10% fetal bovine serum in 2-cm^2 dishes for the specified periods. Erythropoietin was assayed using ^{125}I-labeled recombinant human erythropoietin and antiserum towards recombinant human erythropoietin. The results are given as the mean ± SEM of four to six separate experiments. (Unpublished observations)

Nonrenal Neoplasms

Primary carcinoma of the liver is usually associated with anemia. However, in a review of 340 patients with tumor-induced erythrocytosis, 64 cases of hepatoma were noted [25]. Erythrocytosis occurs in 4% to 12% of all patients with liver carcinoma [37, 43]. Plasma erythropoietin has been shown to be elevated in about 70% of the polycythemic patients [19, 25, 43]. Using a sensitive radioimmunoassay, Kew and Fisher [37] have found an increase in serum erythropoietin in 23% of 65 nonanemic patients with hepatocellular carcinoma. Only one of these was polycythemic. Perhaps bone marrow erythropoiesis was inhibited in most of the patients due to the chronic malignant disease, or the tumor-derived erythropoietin was biologically inactive [37]. Some tissue extracts from liver carcinomas of polycythemic patients exhibited increased erythropoietin bioactivity [25, 46]. Previous attempts to extract erythropoietin from livers of hypoxia-exposed animals without malignancy were unsuccessful [32]. From immunofluorescence and carbon ingestion studies, Gruber et al. [22, 23] earlier suggested that Kupffer cells are the physiological site of the production of erythropoietin in the liver. However, to clarify this point erythropoietin mRNA would need to be demonstrated in a distinct type of liver cells. Okabe et al. [52] have reported erythropoietin release by a hepatocellular carcinoma in primary culture. Recently, it has been shown that cultures of the two established human liver carcinoma cell lines HepG2 and Hep3B produce significant amounts or erythropoietin in culture (Fig. 4) [20, 51]. Thus, it seems likely that liver carcinoma cells synthesize erythropoietin directly, and not indirectly by creating local tissue hypoxia.

Cerebellar hemangioblastoma is found in about 20% of all patients with tumor-associated erythrocytosis [25, 31, 69]. Paraneoplastic erythrocytosis disappeared after removal of the tumor in all of the 26 cases reported by Hammond and Winnick [25]. Recurrence of the tumor was associated with return of erythrocytosis. Very high levels of erythropoietin have been found in the cyst fluid and in extracts of hemangioblastomas, while plasma erythropoietin was usually not elevated [27, 30, 69]. It has been proposed that the determination of the plasma erythropoietin level could provide an aid for the diagnosis and follow-up of patients with hemangioblastomas [2]. Recently, measurements of erythropoietin in the cerebrospinal fluid have been considered to be more reliable here, as high values may be found at low plasma erythropoietin [30]. In immunohistochemical studies with antiserum towards human urinary erythropoietin, positive staining for erythropoietin of scattered "small granular cells" was observed in all hemangioblastomas. The same cells also stained for angiotensinogen and α-1-antitrypsin [4].

Waldmann and Rosse [69] earlier noted that the syndrome von Hippel-Lindau disease includes three tumors which are associated with neoplastic erythrocytosis. Cerebellar hemangioblastoma is found in 47%, renal carcinoma or cysts in 32%, and pheochromocytoma in 14% of the patients [50]. Very few cases have been reported of erythrocytosis in association with pheochromocytoma [69]. Waldmann and Bradley [68] have demonstrated increased erythropoietin activity in the serum and in tumor extracts from a boy with pheochromocytoma.

There have been several reports on erythrocytosis secondary to paraneoplastic production of erythropoietin by smooth muscle tumors [25, 69]. Polycythemia disappeared in 24 of 25 patients after resection of uterine fibromyomata [25]. Plasma erythropoietin was not elevated [25, 49,71] except in a patient studied by Ossias et al. [53]. Cyst fluid and tissue extract of uterine fibromyomas were erythropoietically active [49, 53, 71]. Increased erythropoietin in plasma and tumor extracts was also observed in single cases of leiomyoma of the esophagus [16] and the skin [14]. In addition, a case has been reported of polycythemia and increased serum erythropoietin in association with myxoma of the right atrium [6].

Concluding Remarks

Abnormal erythropoiesis in tumor patients raises a variety of questions of pathophysiological and therapeutic interest. The pathogenesis of the anemia associated with most malignancies displays some similarities to that of other chronic disorders like infection and inflammation. The improvement in immunological techniques will enable investigators to assay erythropoietin more frequently in tumor patients and to provide more precise data, especially in the lower range of plasma erythropoietin levels. From such data, medical priorities may be deduced with regard to the recent possibility of treating anemic patients with recombinant human erythropoietin. For example, recent data from our own laboratory indicate that patients with acute leukemia and severe bone marrow insufficiency have very high plasma levels of erythropoietin. Evidently, there is less need for a replacement therapy in patients with endogenously increased erythropoietin levels. Finally, measurements of erythropoietin may prove useful in the diagnosis and follow-up of malignant diseases associated with erythrocytosis secondary to the production of erythropoietin by neoplasms.

References

1. Altaffer LFW, Chenault OW (1979) Paraneoplastic endocrinopathies associated with renal tumors. J Urol 122: 573–577
2. Anagnostou A, Chawla MS, Pololi L, Fried W (1979) Determination of plasma erythropoietin levels. Cancer 44: 1014–1016
3. Bennett JM, Catovsky D, Daniel MT, Flandrin G, Galton DAG, Gralnick HR, Sultan C (1976) Proposals for the classification of the acute leukaemia. Br J Haematol 33: 451–458
4. Böhling T, Haltia M, Rosenlöf K, Fyhrquist F (1987) Erythropoietin in capillary hemangioblastoma. Acta Neuropathol (Berl) 74: 324–328
5. Bruneval P, da Silva JL, Lacombe C, Salzmann JL, Tambourin P, Varet B, Camilleri JP, Bariety J (1988) Erythropoietin synthesis in the anemic mouse kidney, as observed by morphological techniques. Lübeck Conference on the Pathophysiology and Pharmacology of Erythropoietin, Lübeck, FRG, 25 June
6. Burns ER, Schulman IC, Murphy MJ (1982) Hematologic manifestations and etiology of atrial myxoma. Am J Med Sci 284: 17–22
7. Cartwright GE (1966) The anemia of chronic disorders. Semin Hematol 3: 351–375
8. Cox R, Musial T, Gyde OHB (1986) Reduced erythropoietin levels as a cause of anaemia in patients with lung cancer. Eur J Cancer Clin Oncol 22: 511–514
9. Dainiak N, Kulkarni V, Howard D, Kalmanti M, Dewey MC, Hoffman R (1983) Mechanisms of abnormal erythropoiesis in malignancy. Cancer 51: 1101–1106
10. De Gowin RL, Gibson DP (1979) Erythropoietin and the anemia of mice bearing extramedullary tumor. J Lab Clin Med 94: 303–311
11. Douglas SW, Adamson JW (1975) The anemia of chronic disorders: studies of marrow regulation and iron metabolism. Blood 45: 55–65
12. Eaves AC, Eaves CJ (1979) Abnormalities in the erythroid progenitor compartments in patients with chronic myelogenous leukemia (CML). Exp Hematol 7 [Suppl 5]: 65–75

13. Eaves AC, Eaves CJ (1984) Erythropoiesis in culture. Clin Haematol 13: 371–391
14. Eldor A, Even-Paz Z, Polliack A (1976) Erythrocytosis associated with multiple cutaneous leiomyomata: report of a case with demonstration of erythropoietic activity in the tumour. Scand J Haematol 16: 245–249
15. Firat D, Banzon J (1971) Erythropoietic effect of plasma from patients with advanced cancer. Cancer Res 31: 1353–1359
16. Fried W, Ward HP, Hopeman AR (1968) Leiomyoma and erythrocytosis: a tumor producing a factor which increases erythropoietin production. Report of a case. Blood 31: 813–816
17. Fukushima Y, Miura I, Takahashi T, Fukuda M, Yoshida K, Yamaguchi A, Miura AB (1984) Serum erythropoietin (ESF) levels and erythroid progenitors (CFU–Es) of patients with chronic myeloproliferative disorders. Tohoku J Exp Med 142: 399–407
18. Gabuzda TG, Shute HE, Erslev AJ (1969) Regulation of erythropoiesis in erythroleukemia. Arch Intern Med 123: 60–63
19. Gallagher NI, Donati RM (1968) Inappropriate erythropoietin elaboration. Ann NY Acad Sci 149: 528–538
20. Goldberg MA, Glass GA, Cunningham JM, Bunn HF (1987) The regulated expression of erythropoietin by two human hepatoma cell lines. Proc Natl Acad Sci USA 84: 7972–7976
21. Goldman JM, Shiota F, Th'ng KH, Orchard KH (1980) Circulating granulocytic and erythroid progenitor cells in chronic granulocytic leukaemia. Br J Haematol 46: 7–13
22. Gruber DF, Zucali JR, Wleklinski J, LaRussa V, Mirand EA (1977) Temporal transition in the site of rat erythropoietin production. Exp Hematol 5: 399–407
23. Gruber DF, Zucali JR, Mirand EA (1977) Identification of erythropoietin producing cells in fetal mouse liver cultures. Exp Hematol 5: 392–398
24. Hagiwara M, Chen IL, McGonigle R, Beckman B, Kasten FH, Fisher JW (1984) Erythropoietin production in a primary culture of human renal carcinoma cells maintained in nude mice. Blood 63: 828–835
25. Hammond D, Winnick S (1974) Paraneoplastic erythrocytosis and extopic erythropoietins. Ann NY Acad Sci 230: 219–227
26. Hankins WD, Schooley J, Eastment C (1986) Erythropietin, an autocrine regulator? Serum-free production of erythropoietin by cloned erythroid cell lines. Blood 68: 263–268
27. Hennessy TG, Stern WE, Herrick SE (1967) Cerebellar hemangioblastoma: erythropoietic activity by radioiron assay. J Nucl Med 8: 601–606
28. Hoffman R, Zanjani ED (1978) Erythropoietin dependent erythropoiesis during the erythroblastic phase of juvenile chronic granulocytic leukaemia. Br J Haematol 38: 511–516
29. Hoffman R, Kopel S, Hsu SD, Dainiak N, Zanjani ED (1978) T cell chronic lymphocytic leukemia: presence in bone marrow and peripheral blood of cells that suppress erythropoiesis in vitro. Blood 52: 255–260
30. Jankovic GM, Ristic MS, Pavlovic-Kentera V (1986) Cerebellar hemangioblastoma with erythropoietin in cerebrospinal fluid. Scand J Haematol 36: 511–514
31. Jeffreys RV, Napier JAF, Reynolds SH (1982) Erythropoietin levels in posterior fossa haemangioblastoma. J Neurol Neurosurg Psychiatry 45: 264–266
32. Jelkmann W (1986) Renal erythropoietin: properties and production. Rev Physiol Biochem Pharmacol 104: 139–215
33. Johannsen H, Jelkmann W, Wiedemann G, Otte M, Wagner T (1989) Erythropoietin/haemoglobin relationship in leukaemia and ulcerative colitis. Eur J Haematol (in press)
34. Katsuoko Y, McGonigle R, Rege AB, Beckman B, Fisher JW (1983) Erythropoietin production in human renal carcinoma cells passaged in nude mice and in tissue culture. Gann 74: 534–541
35. Kazal LA, Erslev AJ (1975) Erythropoietin production in renal tumors. Ann Clin Lab Sci 5: 98–109
36. Kenny GM, Mirand EA, Staubitz WJ, Allen JE, Trudel PJ, Murphy GP (1970) Erythropoietin levels in Wilms' tumor patients. J Urol 104: 758–761
37. Kew MC, Fisher JW (1986) Serum erythropoietin concentrations in patients with hepatocellular carcinoma. Cancer 58: 2485–2488

38. Kojima S, Mimaya J, Tonouchi T, Yokochi T, Kajitani S (1987) Erythropoiesis during an erythroblastic phase of chronic myeloproliferative disorder associated with monosomy 7. Br J Haematol 65: 391–394
39. Koury ST, Bondurant MC, Koury MJ (1988) Localization of erythropoietin synthesizing cells in murine kidneys by in situ hybridization. Blood 71: 524–527
40. Kurnick JE, Ward HP, Pickett JC (1972) Mechanism of the anemia of chronic disorders. Arch Intern Med 130: 323–326
41. Kvarstein B, Lindemann R, Mathisen W (1973) Renal carcinoma with increased erythropoietin production and secondary polycythemia. Scand J Urol Nephrol 7: 178–180
42. Lan S, McCulloch EA, Till JA (1978) Cytodifferentiation in the acute myeloblastic leukemias of man. J Natl Cancer Inst 60: 265–269
43. McFadzean AJS, Todd D, Tso SC (1967) Erythrocytosis associated with hepatocellular carcinoma. Blood 29: 808–811
44. Lacombe C, Da Silva JL, Bruneval P, Fournier JG, Wendling F, Casadevall N, Camilleri JP, Bariety J, Varet B, Tambourin P (1988) Peritubular cells are the site of erythropietin synthesis in the murine hypoxic kidney. J Clin Invest 81: 620–623
45. Morse EE (1979) Consequences of erythropoietin production by neoplasms. Ann Clin Lab Sci 9: 116–120
46. Murphy GP, Mirand EA (1971) Erythropoietin alterations in human renal disease. Rev Surg 28: 236–245
47. Murphy GP, Mirand EA, Johnston GS, Gibbons RP, Jones RL, Scott WW (1967) Erythropoietin release associated with Wilms' tumor. Johns Hopkins Med J 120: 26–32
48. Murphy GP, Mirand EA, Staubitz WJ (1976) The value of erythropoietin assay in the follow-up of Wilms' tumor patients. Oncology 33: 154–156
49. Naets JP, Wittek M, Delwiche F, Kram I (1977) Polycythaemia and erythropoietin producing uterine fibromyoma. Scand J Haematol 19: 75–78
50. Neumann HPH (1987) Basic criteria for clinical diagnosis and genetic counselling in von Hippel-Lindau syndrome. VASA 16: 220–226
51. Nielsen OJ, Schuster SJ, Kaufman R, Erslev AJ, Caro J (1987) Regulation of erythropoietin production in a human hepatoblastoma cell line. Blood 70: 1904–1909
52. Okabe T, Urabe A, Kato T, Chiba S, Takaku F (1985) Production of erythropoietin-like activity by human renal and hepatic carcinomas in cell culture. Cancer 55: 1918–1923
53. Ossias AL, Zanjani ED, Zalusky R, Estren S, Wasserman LR (1973) Case report: studies on the mechanism of erythrocytosis associated with a uterine fibromyoma. Br J Haematol 25: 179–185
54. Pavlovic-Kentera V, Stefanovic S, Milenkovic P, Jancic M, Biljanovic-Paunovic L (1976) Erythropoietin level in patients with acute leukaemia. Haematologia (Budap) 10: 455–462
55. Roodman GD (1987) Mechanisms of erythroid suppression in the anemia of chronic disease. Blood Cells 13: 171–184
56. Schooley JC, Kullgren B, Allison AC (1987) Inhibition by interleukin-1 of the action of erythropoietin on erythroid precursors and its possible role in the pathogenesis of hypoplastic anaemias. Br J Haematol 67: 11–17
57. Schreuder WO, Ting WC, Smith S, Jacobs A (1984) Testosterone, erythropoietin and anaemia in patients with disseminated bronchial cancer. Br J Haematol 57: 521–526
58. Shalet MF, Holder TM, Walters TR (1967) Erythropoietin-producing Wilms' tumor. J Pediatr 70: 615–617
59. Shalhoub RJ, Rajan U, Kim VV, Goldwasser E, Kark JA, Antoniou LD (1982) Erythrocytosis in patients on long-term hemodialysis. Ann Intern Med 97: 686–690
60. Sherwood JB, Goldwasser E (1976) Erythropoietin production by human renal carcinoma cells in culture. Endocrinology 99: 504–510
61. Slee PHTJ, Blusse A, Brutel de la Riviere G, den Ottolander GJ (1978) Erythrocytosis and Wilms' tumour. Scand J Haematol 21: 287–291
62. Sufrin G, Mirand EA, Moore RH, Chu TM, Murphy GP (1977) Hormones in renal cancer. J Urol 117: 433–438

63. Sytkowski AJ, Bicknell KA, Smith GM, Garcia JF (1984) Secretion of erythropoietin-like acitivity by clones of human renal carcinoma cell line GKA. Cancer Res 44: 51–54
64. Thorling EB (1965) Erythropoietin in serum from patients with leucosis assays in starved rats. Scand J Haematol 2: 36–51
65. Thorling EB (1972) Paraneoplastic erythrocytosis and inappropriate erythropoietin production. Scand J Haematol 17: 1–166
66. Toogood IRG, Ekert H, Smith PJ (1978) Controlled study of hypertransfusion during remission induction in childhood acute lymphocytic leukaemia. Lancet ii: 862–864
67. Toyama K, Fujiyama N, Suzuki H, Chen TP, Tamaoki N, Ueyama Y (1979) Erythropoietin levels in the course of a patient with erythropoietin-producing renal cell carcinoma and transplantation of this tumor in nude mice. Blood 54: 245–253
68. Waldmann TA, Bradley JE (1961) Polycythemia secondary to a pheochromocytoma with production of an erythropoiesis stimulating factor by the tumor. Proc Soc Exp Biol Med 108: 425–427
69. Waldmann TA, Rosse W (1964) Tumors producing erythropoiesis-stimulating factors. In: Sundermann FW, Sundermann FW (eds) Hemoglobin, its precursors and metabolites. Lippincott, Philadelphia, pp 276–280
70. Ward HP, Kurnick JE, Pisarczyk MJ (1971) Serum level of erythropoietin in anemias associated with chronic infection, malignancy, and primary hematopoietic disease. J Clin Invest 50: 332–335
71. Wrigley PFM, Malpas JS, Turnbull AL, Jenkins GC, McArt A (1971) Secondary polycythaemia due to a uterine fibromyoma producing erythropoietin. Br J Haematol 21: 551–555
72. Zucker S, Friedman S, Lysik RM (1974) Bone marrow erythropoiesis in the anemia of infection, inflammation, and malignancy. J Clin Invest 53: 1132–1138

Pathophysiology of Erythropoiesis in Renal Diseases*

V. PAVLOVIĆ-KENTERA, G. K. CLEMONS, and L. DJUKANOVIĆ

The role of erythropoietin in the regulation of erythropoiesis is well documented. Conclusive evidence exists that the kidney is a major source of erythropoietin. Not surprisingly, anemia or secondary erythrocytosis accompanies renal diseases. Anemia is a regular feature of chronic renal failure and its primary cause is decreased erythropoietin production, while secondary erythrocytosis is caused by increased erythropoietin.

Anemia in Chronic Renal Failure

Anemia in chronic renal failure is the most consistent feature contributing significantly to the morbidity of this disease. It was recognized by Bright as a complication of uremia back in 1836 [48]. The severity of uremic anemia depends on the impairment of renal function. However, different levels of anemia are found in patients with the same degree of renal failure. Regular hemodialysis or continuous ambulatory peritoneal dialysis to relieve patients of uremic symptoms does not cure their anemia.

The mechanism of anemia in chronic renal failure is a complex ohne [31]. Shortened red cell survival, decreased erythropoietin production, inhibition of erythropoiesis by inhibitors present in uremic sera, iron and folic acid deficiencies and protein malnutrition are factors of varying importance in the etiology of anemia in chronic renal failure. However, the principal factor in this anemia is insufficient erythropoietin production. Correction of the anemia with human erythropoietin has confirmed the importance of erythropoietin deficiency in the pathogenesis of the anemia of chronic renal failure [29, 108].

---

* This study was supported by a grant from the Serbian Research Foundation. The research was also supported in part by a grant from the National Heart, Lung and Blood Institute (NHLBI-22469), USA, and conducted at the Lawrence Berkeley Laboratory (Department of Energy contract DE-AC03-76SF00098 to the University of California).

Red Cell Survival

One of the mechanisms implicated in the anemia of chronic renal failure is increased red blood cell (RBC) destruction [52]. Although in renal failure increased hemolysis is typical, it is only a moderate increase and should be easily compensated by a normal erythroid marrow [27]. The RBC life span in these patients is shortened to approximately half the normal life span [30]. This hemolysis seems to be due to extracorpuscular factors and not to any intracorpuscular defect of the erythrocytes, since the transfusion of a patient's red cells into normal persons normalizes RBC survival while the reverse procedure shortens the life span of the transfused cells [45]. The shortened RBC life span is attributed to interference by an unidentified substance in uremic plasma with the function of Na^+/K^+-dependent ATPase [37]. A role for methylguanidine in the shortened RBC life span in uremia has been postulated [31]. RBC survival is not improved either by hemodialysis or continuous peritoneal dialysis [27].

In some uremic patients an RBC metabolic abnormality which diminishes the activity of the pentose phosphate shunt has been found [110]. It has been suggested that the inefficient phosphoglyceromutase activity underlying this abnormality is due to a circulating partial inhibitor of the enzyme [110]. The abnormality in the pentose phosphate shunt causes impaired NADPH generation and reduced glutathione, thereby increasing RBC susceptibility to oxidative stress [44].

Splenomegaly is a common finding in patients on maintenance hemodialysis. A hypersplenic syndrome with increased RBC destruction develops only in some patients on maintenance hemodialysis and contributes to the severity of the patient's anemia. Hypersplenism is probably immunologic in nature and a consequence of repeated antigen stimulation. Splenectomy reduces the need for blood transfusions, although an improvement in RBC survival has not been seen to follow [4].

A characteristic finding in uremic anemia is the presence on peripheral blood smears of echinocytes. Their number has shown no correlation with the severity ot the anemia. This morphological abnormality is probably the consequence of some humoral factor present in uremic serum [1]. There are suggestions that the echinocytes in uremia are, at least in part, artifactual and do not circulate in the blood [26].

There is no impairment of the oxygen carrying capacity of red blood cells in uremia. The concentration of 2,3-diphosphoglycerate increases in response to anemia and hyperphosphatemia, and the affinity of hemoglobin for oxygen decreases correspondingly. The ability of uremic erythrocytes to release oxygen to the body tissues is thereby enhanced. The stimulus for erythropoietin production may the reduced by the improved oxygen delivery to the tissues, but improved oxygen delivery also improves tolerance of anemia in uremic patients. The question is what level of anemia is adequate for satisfactory tissue oxygenation in these patients. It has been suggested that the anemia of stable uremia is an adaptive process for bringing a greater plasma volume into contact with the diminished glomerular filtering surface. A lower hematocrit would increase the efficiency of this process [1].

Erythropoietin

Decreased bone marrow stimulation by erythropoietin in the anemia associated with renal failure was recognized 30 years ago [39]. Serum erythropoietin levels in patients with renal failure were thought to be below the normal values because at the time the only possibility for detecting erythropoietin in biological fluids was by indirect determination in starved or polycythemic rats [51], and later in polycythemic mice. Just as for most normal persons, for most anemic patients with chronic renal failure serum erythropoietin levels remained undetectable by these low sensitivity in vivo assays ([48, 67] an others). Slightly increased serum erythropoietin levels were nevertheless found by means of these bioassays in a few patients [30, 60, 68, 81, 94, 113]. One study was an exception in its results [20]. When a plasma concentration technique was used by Caro et al. [8], measurable serum erythropoietin levels were obtained for normal persons and uremic patients by mouse assay. It was then found that in a group of nephric patients on maintenance hemodialysis, eight had serum erythropoietin levels in the range of the normal nonuremic controls while six had higher than normal serum erythropoietin levels. The increased erythropoietin levels found in these patients with end-stage renal failure were below the erythropoietin levels of patients with a comparable degree of anemia and normal renal function. In the same study, serum erythropoietin levels in eight of 11 anephric patients were detectable but very low.

A sensitive in vitro assay – the fetal mouse liver cell bioassay – has also been used to measure erythropoietin levels in patients with anemia and renal diseases. The results obtained are important, but the specificity of this in vitro assay is questioned. In predialysis patients at various stages of renal insufficiency and with anemia, serum erythropoietin levels were found to be slightly elevated [76]. In nephric patients on regular hemodialysis and with a comparable degree of anemia, serum erythropoietin levels were in the range of normal values [46]. In anephric patients, erythropoietin levels were lower than those of the normal controls [78]. With a modification of the same assay, the results obtained by de Klerk et al. [21] differed. The mean erythropoietin concentration values found for both uremic patients in the predialysis stage and patients on maintenance hemodialysis were significantly below normal. A considerable overlap of serum erythropoietin values for the two patients groups and the normal controls was, however present. In patients on maintenance hemodialysis a positive correlation between serum erythropoietin level and hemoglobin concentration was found [21]. In children with chronic renal failure on conservative treatment, serum erythropoietin levels similar to those of healthy children and higher than for children on maintenance hemodialysis were found by a modified in vitro assay [65].

Although different absolute values were obtained by the different authors using modifications of the fetal mouse liver assay, it seems important that overall their results indicate a low but quantitatively normal erythropoietin response to anemia in predialysis patients, that is, sustained regulatory feedback mechanism between hematocrit and serum erythropoietin level [76].

Radioimmunoassay has been used to measure serum erythropoietin level in patients with renal diseases since this technique was developed by investigators [16, 40, 88].

A large group of 60 patients not receiving any form of dialysis treatment and with hematocrit values ranging from 16.5% to 52% was studied by McGonigle et al. [55]. Erythropoietin levels were determined by the radioimmunoassay developed at their institution [82]. Increased serum levels of immunoreactive erythropoietin were found in seven out of these 60 patients with varying degrees of renal insufficiency. The other erythropoietin values were within the normal range. Serum erythropoietin levels showed no relationship to plasma creatinine, hematocrit or the serum level of uremic inhibitors for any patient. Similar findings were obtained in 31 children with renal disease of different origins and varying severity. In the four anephric children in whom anemia was most severe, serum erythropoietin levels were significantly lower than in the normal controls [54].

We have investigated anemia in groups of predialysis patients at different stages of renal failure due to three underlying diseases: Balkan endemic nephropathy (BEN), chronic pyelonephritis and glomerulonephritis. The study of a total of 88 patients focussed on whether a correlation exists between the severity of anemia and the stage of renal failure, and whether erythropoietin production depends on the type and stage of nephropathy. Of particular interest was the anemia in BEN, a tubulointerstitial nephropathy [18]. It had been claimed that in BEN anemia precedes renal failure [19]. The postulated cause would be a the early damage of erythropoietin-producing kidney cells defined by Schuster et al. [84] and by Lacombe et al. [49]. The results are presented in Tables 1 and 2.

Significant positive correlation between creatinine clearance and hemoglobin concentration was found in all three nephropathies, indicating that the severity of anemia increased with the impairment of renal function regardless of the underlying disease. The patients had hemoglobin concentrations from 70 to 160 g/l. Serum immunoreactive erythropoietin levels were in the normal range in 54, moderately increased in 20, and only slightly decreased in 14 cases. The erythropoietin level appears to be unrelated to the degree of azotemia or the type of nephropathy. The only exception is subgroup 1, were the patients with glomerulonephritis and normal renal function had increased serum erythropoietin levels and significantly higher RBC parameters than the patients in this subgroup with tubulointerstitial nephropathies. A weak negative correlation between serum erythropoietin levels and hemoglobin concentrations was found only in patients with glomerulonephirits, indicating normal feedback regulation of erythropoietin production in these patients.

Cotes [15] reported that in 22 nephric patients with anemia and on maintenance hemodialysis, serum immunoreactive erythropoietin levels were found to be in the range of the normal controls and lower than in patients with a similar degree of "non-renal" anemia. In eight anephric patients serum immunoreactive erythropoietin was detectable, but at lower levels, and essentially unrelated to the severity of anemia. In 11 hemodialysis patients with varying degrees of anemia, serum

Table 1. Sex, age and creatinine clearance in predialysis patients with different nephropathies

Sub-group	BEN				PN				GN				Ccr (ml/min)		
	n	Sex M	F	Age (years)	*n*	Sex M	F	Age (years)	*n*	Sex M	F	Age (years)	BEN	PN	GN
1	8	3	5	60.8 ± 7.8	5	2	3	52.2 ± 9.0	5	4	1	39.2* ± 10.8	98 ± 12.9	99 ± 8.4	99.6 ± 7.1
2	9	6	3	65.1 ± 7.6	5	1	4	45.8* ± 15.9	5	4	1	40.2* ± 10.3	58.9 ± 6.2	69.8 ± 11.1	67.4 ± 9.9
3	18	8	10	63.4 ± 10.8	5	0	5	52 ± 12.2	5	4	1	41.2* ± 14.7	31.7 ± 6.3	38.2 ± 7.6	30.6 ± 8.3
4	13	5	8	65.8 ± 8.1	5	2	3	66.6 ± 4.8	5	4	1	55.8 ± 14.2	12.8 ± 5.3	17.0 ± 3.7	15.6 ± 4.3

Age and creatinine clearance (Ccr) expressed as mean ± SD
BEN, Balkan endemic nephropathy; PN, pyelonephritis; GN, glomerulonephritis
* Significantly different from BEN ($p < 0.05$)

Table 2. Measures of red cell concentration and serum level of immunoreactive erythropoietin in the patients studied

Subgroup	Red cells (× 10^{12}/l) BEN	PN	GN	Hematocrit (%) BEN	PN	GN	Hemoglobin (g/l) BEN	PN	GN	Erythropoietin (mU/ml) BEN	PN	GN
1	3.90 ± 0.38	4.01 ± 0.25	4.49*+ ± 0.25	39.5 ± 3.8	42.6 ± 1.9	45.6* ± 2.7	134 ± 14.5	135.8 ± 13.2	141*+ ± 16.2	18.6 ± 1.5	19.7 ± 4.1	44.1*+ ± 20.4
2	3.71 ± 0.50	4.13 ± 0.58	4.01 ± 0.65	37.6 ± 5.2	40.8 ± 4.4	40.8 ± 5.7	127 ± 21.3	133.2 ± 17.3	124.4 ± 21.0	21.3 ± 8.4	17.0 ± 4.9	16.9 ± 0.6
3	3.35 ± 0.41	3.02 ± 0.45	2.72* ± 0.24	33.6 ± 4.0	30.0 ± 3.7	26.2* ± 2.7	111.7 ± 18.7	93.6 ± 15.5	85.4* ± 9.1	17.5 ± 3.8	23.0* ± 6.8	16.4 ± 2.4
4	2.52 ± 0.54	2.79 ± 0.57	2.69 ± 0.25	25.2 ± 5.4	28.8 ± 4.8	26.4 ± 1.8	84.4 ± 16.7	89.8 ± 18.6	84.6 ± 4.7	19.4 ± 4.9	31.1 ± 25.5	23.7 ± 16.0
p 2 : 3		< 0.001	< 0.001		< 0.001	< 0.001		< 0.001	< 0.001			
p 3 : 4	< 0.001			< 0.001			< 0.001					

Data expressed as mean ± SD
BEN, Balkan endemic nephropathy; PN, pyelonephritis; GN, glomerulonephritis
* Significantly different from BEN ($p < 0.05$)
+ Significantly different from PN ($p < 0.05$)

immunoreactive erythropoietin levels from normal to slightly above normal were reported by Zaroulis et al [112].

Similar serum erythropoietin concentrations were found in 46 patients receiving regular hemodialysis (mean hematocrit value 25.9% ± 1.4%) and 30 patients on continuous ambulatory peritoneal dialysis (mean hematocrit value 30.4% ± 1.3%). Serum immunoreactive erythropoietin levels were found to be above the normal range but inappropriately low for the degree of anemia. No significant difference was seen in the mean erythropoietin values between the two groups of dialysis patients. Serum erythropoietin concentrations were not related to hematocrit changes in the patients receiving continuous ambulatory peritoneal dialysis, and were no higher in patients with polycystic kidney disease than in patients with end-stage renal disease due to other causes [57].

In another study, serum immunoreactive erythropoietin values in 21 anemic nephric and anephric patients on maintenance hemodialysis did not differ from the normal controls. The erythropoietin levels in this patient group showed no relationship to the severity of anemia [66]. Radioimmunoassay was used also by Urabe et al. [99] to determine the serum erythropoietin levels of 17 patients. All the patients were anemic and on maintenance hemodialysis. The erythropoietin levels found were lower than those in a patient group with iron deficiency anemia and comparable hemoglobin concentrations (5 to 10 g/dl).

Serum immunoreactive erythropoietin levels were measured by Chandra et al. [12] in two groups of patients on maintenance hemodialysis: patients with autosomal dominant polycistic kidney disease and patients with other kidney diseases. The erythropoietin levels of the 12 patients with polycystic kidney disease did not differ from the normal control values but were higher than in the patients with other kidney diseases whose erythropoietin values were significantly lower than in the normal controls. Similar results were obtained by Pavlović-Kentera et al. [73] with the same radioimmunoassay. Although higher erythropoietin levels were found for patients with polycystic kidney disease on maintenance hemodialysis, these accorded with the higher hematocrits obtained in this patients group.

Others have reported [41] and we have also noted that patients on maintenance hemodialysis show an improvement in their anemia. The improvement, however, differs significantly among hemodialysed patients. In order to investigate the differences in the pathophysiology of erythropoiesis in anemic and nonanemic patients who had been on maintenance hemodialysis for more than 1 year we formed and studied three groups of patients: anemic patients with hematocrit values < 20% (group A) and two subgroups of nonanemic patients with hematocrit values > 30% – those with polycystic kidney disease (group PKD) and those with other nephropathies (group NA). In Table 3 relevant data for patients from groups A, NA and PKD are presented. The main difference between the three patient groups was in their serum immunoreactive erythropoietin level at the time of the study. Patients with polycystic kidney disease had high serum erythropoietin levels, as we expected on the basis of our earlier work [73]. In patients with other kidney diseases whose anemia improved after a period on maintenance hemodialysis erythropoietin levels were moderately increased, while in patients whose anemia

Table 3. Red blood cell concentration parameters, serum level of iron (Fe), transferrin and immunoreactive erythropoietin (Ep) and the duration of hemodialysis (HD) in patients with end-stage renal disease

Group	n	HD (months)	RBC ($\times 10^{12}$/l)	Ht (%)	Hb (g/l)	Iron (μmol/l)	Transferrin (g/l)	Ep (mU/ml)	ACKD (n)
A	14	67.1* ± 47.7	1.78* ± 0.31	18.1* ± 2.9	58.1* ± 9.5	16.2 ± 4.5	2.5* ± 0.4	20.0* ± 4.4	5
NA	14	100.9 ± 40.8	3.61 ± 0.45	36.7 ± 4.0	114.4 ± 13.0	13.8 ± 5.0	3.3 ± 1.0	26.2 ± 8.6	11
PKD	9	55.7 ± 38.0	3.72 ± 0.66	38.2 ± 7.0	121.7 ± 23.2	10.0* ± 3.8	3.1 ± 0.2	142.8* ± 152.7	

Data expressed as mean ± SD
A, anemic patients; NA, nonanemic patients; PKD, nonanemic patients with polycystic kidney disease; Ht, hematocrit; Hb, hemoglobin; ACKD, acquired cystic kidney disease
* Significantly different from other two groups ($p < 0.05$)

showed no improvement erythropoietin levels were in the normal range, i. e., inappropriately low for the degree of their anemia. The differences in serum erythropoietin levels in the patients investigated here confirms the importance of erythropoietin deficiency in the anemia of chronic renal failure. The relationship between serum erythropoietin and hematocrit levels calculated for all the patients studied was positive, contrary to the well-known inverse relationship in anemic patients without kidney disease.

Although radioimmunoassay for erythropoietin made available a useful tool for investigating the pathophysiology of erythropoiesis in chronic renal failure, a question has been raised concerning the validity of results obtained by immunoassay [27]. The point must be made here that every immunoassay reported had been validated [13, 15, 25, 82]. This does not exclude the possibility of the presence of a substance devoid of biological activity but with the same characteristics as erythropoietin in its immunological reaction [88, 89]. Recombinant erythropoietin-derived reagents will now enable the broader use of radioimmunoassay. Patients with different degrees of renal insufficiency can be followed up [25] and data of greater significance obtained.

Erythropoietin levels measured by radioimmunoassays have given, despite the relatively small patients groups involved, important results. It has been demonstrated that anemia in chronic renal failure develops as renal function deteriorates when serum erythropoietin level remains unchanged. When higher than normal erythropoietin values have been found, the patients were either nonanemic or had mild anemia. Anephric patients have the most severe anemia, and their erythropoietin levels have been below normal. These findings confirm that the most important factor in the pathogenesis of anemia in chronic renal failure is the insufficient production of erythropoietin.

It needs to be stressed that in the sera of some patients with no residual excretory kidney function, high erythropoietin levels have been measured, indicating the retention by kidney tissue of its endocrine function. However, direct proof of renal as opposed to extrarenal erythropoietin production has not always been found. That a diseased kidney can sustain erythropoietin secretion was demonstrated by Dagher et al. [17] for a patient with a kidney allograft where erythropoietin levels were higher in the renal venous plasma of the original diseased kidney than of the transplanted kidney. Further findings include the development of erythrocytosis in patients with end-stage renal failure and on maintenance hemodialysis [86] and the reported nephrectomized transplanted patient whose graft kidney was capable of functioning as an erythropoietin-producing organ despite the loss of excretory function [9].

The positive correlation between the hematocrit values and serum erythropoietin levels found in patient groups with end-stage renal disease and on maintenance hemodialysis [21, 65, 73, 77] has suggested that erythropoietin synthesis is not regulated by general hypoxia. Deficient feedback regulation of erythropoietin production in kidney transplant patients with polycythemia was studied by Thevenod et al. [96]. Normal feedback regulation was found for transplanted kidneys but not for native diseased kidneys. It was suggested that erythropoietin production in a diseased kidney either escapes feedback regulation or the feedback mechanism operates only at a higher hemoglobin level.

A full evaluation of these findings is made difficult by the following observations: an anephric patient whose erythropoietin could only be extrarenal showed an erythropoietin level increase from 5 to 99 mU/ml in association with a hemoglobin drop from 5.0 to 3.5 g/dl [15]; in anemic nephric and anephric patients, hematocrit increases observed after transfusion were followed in nearly all the patients by a decrease in serum erythropoietin levels [21, 66]; higher serum immunoreactive erythropoietin levels and reticulocyte counts have been demonstrated in regularly hemodialyzed patients showing hematocrit decreases resulting from spontaneaous hemorrhage, while lower erythropoietin values and reticulocyte counts have been obtained following transfusion [102]. These observations point to the conclusion that the erythropoietin-hematocrit feedback loop persists and that the erythropoietin production is to a certain degree dependent on tissue hypoxia in patients with diseased kidneys or without kidneys [66, 76, 102].

The role of insufficient erythropoietin production as a major cause of anemia in patients with renal failure has been illustrated in some patients on maintenance hemodialysis who contracted hepatitis B during dialysis treatment [14, 47]. A transient improvement of anemia lasting for a few months with an hemoglobin increase high enough to allow regular transfusions to be suspended was described. These finings point to an increase of erythropoietin production by the damaged and regenerating liver similarly to this found in experimental animals [2, 36]. The bilaterally nephrectomized patients included in these patients groups provide especially convincing evidence [7, 14, 47, 75, 90]. Serum erythropoietin levels measured in a limited number of patients on maintenance hemodialysis during periods of liver enzyme abnormality were found to be increased [6, 58]. After tests had confirmed improved liver function, erythropoietin levels were measured and had returned to their previous low values. During the period of liver enzyme abnormality, increased reticulocyte counts and high hemoglobin values showed that the bone marrow of these patients was responding to the elevated erythropoietin level despite the uremic milieu. It is most unfortunate that only a damaged and regenerating liver regains some of its fetal capacity to secrete erythropoietin and that this organ does not take over when kidneys are damaged or absent.

Erythropoiesis Inhibitors

The role of erythropiesis inhibitors in the anemia of chronic renal failure was suggested by Markson and Rennie [53]. They demonstrated the inhibitory effect of azotemic serum in a suspension culture on normoblast maturation. The relative insensitivity of the bone marrow to erythropoietin action in the presence of uremic plasma containing inhibitors has been suggested [5, 100]. McGonigle et al. [54] reported that coincubation of human urinary erythropoietin and uremic serum markedly diminished erythropoietin immunoreactivity and erythropoietin biological activity. Many investigators have reported efforts to clarify this issue, but the importance of specific erythropoiesis inhibitors in the development of anemia in renal failure remains uncertain.

In vitro methods are used to detected erythropiesis inhibitors in the sera of patients with anemia of renal failure. Various cell culture systems are in use. In vivo assays are not used because of the possible ability of animals with normal renal function to excrete the inhibitors. Uremic sera added to bone marrow cultures have been demonstrated to inhibit heme [32, 63, 72, 106]. The inhibition of DNA synthesis in short-term bone marrow cultures has also been reported [42]. The growth of erythroid progenitors from murine and human bone marrow in semisolid media with exogenous erythropoietin added was inhibited by addition of uremic sera [22, 33, 34, 54, 70, 73, 74, 103, 105]. However, lack of specificity of inhibitors for erythropoiesis was reported by Delwishe et al. [22]. Their findings included inhibition of granulocytes and megakaryocytes progenitors in vitro as well, in contrast to the results of McGonigle et al. [54] and Pavlović-Kentera et al. [74]. The importance of inhibitors in uremic anemia was suggested by the finding that sera from patients with the lowest hematocrits were the most inhibitory to in vitro heme synthesis and erythroid colony growth [57, 69, 104]. We found no correlations between the inhibition of in vitro mouse CFU-E growth and the severity of anemia in patients on maintenance hemodialysis [74]. However, for CFU-E growth the percentage of inhibition did depend on serum concentration in cultures. No correlation could be found between serum concentrations of urea, creatinine, uric acid and parathyroid homone and the inhibition of CFU-E growth. A significant linear correlation between inhibition of CFU-E growth and the concentration of certain middle molecular mass serum fractions was seen. Uremic serum fractions and normal human urine fractions obtained in the peak 7 and the peak 4 of gel filtration on Sephadex G-15 [38] significantly inhibited mouse CFU-E growth, while other fractions showed no influence [23].

One suggestion is that erythropoiesis inhibitors might act on erythroid stem cells in anemic uremic patients. However, erythroid progenitors from patients with end-stage renal disease grown in vitro indicated the presence of BFU-E in peripheral blood in adequate number and a normal response to erythropoietin stimulus of these early progenitors removed from the uremic environments [33]. More recently published papers report decreased BFU-E concentrations in the bone marrow [50] and in the peripheral blood [64]. Further investigation is needed of the suggestion of Lamperi and Carozi [50] that a blockage occurs in uremic patients of the interaction between immunocompetent and bone marrow cells required for normal stimulation of early erythroid progenitors. The presence or absence in uremic sera of inhibitors of lymphokines, for instance, should be established.

Various factors present in the sera of anemic patients with chronic renal failure have been implicated as erythropiesis inhibitors. Lipids [103] and low molecular weight polypeptide [42] have been singled out, and excess blood levels of parathyroid hormone have been attributed partial responsibility for this anemia [59]. Investigations of the effect of the parathyroid hormone on erythropoiesis have not produced consistent results. McGonigle et al. [56] were unable to find a significant relationship between serum parathyroid hormone levels and either anemia or the inhibition of erythropoiesis in uremic patients. Spermine and spermidine have proved clearly inhibitory for erythroid colony growth, and antispermine antiserum effectively neutralized the inhibitory effect of uremic serum on erythroid colony growth [80]. The pathophysiologic significance of spermine and spermidine inhibition of erythroid colony growth was questioned by the authors [85] who found that these polyamines also inhibited CFU-GM and CFU-Mk colony growth, and were unable to overcome these inhibitions with specific stimulators (Ep and CSF). Inhibitory uremic serum showed strikingly increased ribonuclease activity, and purified ribonuclease produced dose-dependent inhibition of erythroid colony growth, but a relationship between serum ribonuclease activity and patients' hematocrit values could not be established [35]. Fractionating uremic sera on Sephacryl gel, Freedman et al. [33] located inhibitory activity for erythroid colony growth in the fractions of molecular weights from 47000 to 150000.

Several lines of evidence point to the responsibility of uremic inhibitors for the relative insensitivity of erythroid stem cells to the action of erythropoietin in azotemic patients. The anephric patient described by Ortega et al. [71] illustrated the possible importance of erythropoiesis inhibitors. He was severely anemic and transfusion dependent and yet showed exceptionally high serum erythropoietin biological activity. In vitro his serum clearly inhibited erythropoietin-stimulated erythropoiesis by normal human marrow cells. Additional evidence is the anemia of end-stage renal disease even in the patients with higher than normal erythropoietin levels. Removal of some of erythropoiesis inhibitors could explain the improvement of anemia in patients on maintenance hemodialysis [30, 79] or peritoneal dialysis when there is no change in the level of circulating erythropoietin. Continuous ambulatory peritoneal dialysis has been demonstrated to be more efficient than hemodialysis in the removal fo "middle molecules" implicated as erythropoietin inhibitors and therefore more effective in the improvement of anemia of end-stage renal disease [111]. The results reviewed here indicate the presence in uremic serum of several inhibitors, some too large in molecular size for removal by either form of dialysis.

On the other hand an accumulation of data denies the role of uremic inhibitors as a major contributing factor to the anemia of renal failure. Mladenovic et al. [62], using an autologous sheep model, could find no significant in vitro inhibition by uremic sheep serum. Sera from recombinant erythropoietin-treated hemodialyzed patients failed to suppress in vitro erythroid progenitor growth despite the persistence of a uremic state [109]. The improvement reported recently of the anemia in a patient with end-stage renal disease after the initiation of continuous ambulatory peritoneal dialysis was accompanied by an increased erythropoietin level [11], indicating that the better milieu was provided by peritoneal dialysis for erythropoietin production. Increased plasma erythropoietin levels after initiating peritoneal dialysis had earlier been reported by Winderoë et al. [107].

Conclusive proof that the inhibitors of erythropoiesis are pathogenetic in the anemia of renal failure, even now, after uniform correction of anemia with recombinant human erythropoietin in patients requiring maintenance hemodialysis, remains elusive [29, 108]. The bone marrow of azotemic patients would seem able to respond, despite the presence of inhibitors in the plasma, to erythropoietic stimulus when that stimulus is sufficiently intense.

Iron Metabolism

The anemia in chronic renal failure is usually normocytic and normochromic. Iron deficiency and microcytosis are not common in patients still on conservative treatment. This is because erythropoiesis in the bone marrow decreases and iron absorption from the diet remains normal [28]. Patients with occult gastrointestinal bleeding or bleeding from other sources are the exception. The decrease in hemoglobin level associated with decrease of erythrocyte mean corpusculat volume is usually a late consequence of iron deficiency. In the nondialyzed uremic patients a shift occurs of iron from erythrocytes to iron stores. As renal insufficiency progresses, erythropoiesis decreases and iron stores become elevated [27]. In nontransfused patients on maintenance hemodialysis iron deficiency becomes common owing to the small repetitive blood losses in the dialysis system during hemodialysis, frequent blood sampling for laboratory tests and accidental blood leaks. Iron deficiency is caused by the estimated iron losses of 1.5–2.0 g per year in regularly hemodialyzed patients [28] and can be predicted by measuring the serum ferritin level.

When iron stores are decreased iron supplementation is necessary. This is particularly so when erythropoiesis is stimulated by erythropoietin. Oral iron supplementation is physiological and best for patients with renal failure. The regulation of iron absorption from the gastrointestinal tract will respond to the body's iron stores [28]. When iron stores are increased, iron absorption decreases and iron overload is avoided.

Aluminum Toxicity

Microcytic anemia occurring in patients on maintenance hemodialysis when their iron stores are normal or elevated is described as an aluminum toxicity-related disorder. The mechanism by which aluminum induces microcytic anemia is not known, but an inhibition of hemoglobin synthesis similar to that seen in lead poisoning is suggested [95]. It is known that aluminum interferes in vitro with peroxidase and with deltaaminolevulinic acid dehydrogenase [98]. An explanation for the toxic effect of aluminum on erythron would seem important, particularly from the standpoint of a possible interference with erythropoiesis in the bone marrow stimulated by erythropoietin [27].

Folic Acid and Other Deficiency

Folate deficiency can contribute to anemia in patients on maintenance hemodialysis. Folic acid is dialyzable and small amounts are always lost during dialysis. When the dialysis loss exceeds the dietary intake macrocytosis may develop. This is seen in patients on restricted dietary protein intake or in patients treated with drugs which impair intestinal folate absorption. Patients on an adequate diet usually fully compensate the loss of folate by dialysis [27].

Changes in metabolism and in endocrine function may contribute to the pathogenesis of the anemia of uremia. Protein metabolism abnormalities in patients with chronic renal failure can suppress erythropoietin production in much the same way as does inadequate protein intake [10]. Protein deprivation, like starvation, suppresses erythropoietin production. Endocrine changes could also be attributed to altered protein metabolism in uremic patients [1].

Effect of Enzymes

Increased plasma glucosidase and protease activity has recently been described in patients on maintenance hemodialysis [87]. It was postulated that a combined attack by both these enzymes on erythropoietin may lead to fragmentation of the molecule and its loss of activity. The importance of this increased enzyme activity with regard to possible erythropoietin degradation when erythropoietin is being used to treat the anemia in uremic patients needs further clarification.

Erythrocytosis in Renal Diseases

Secondary erythrocytosis may be seen in the course of a number of renal diseases. It is a consequence of inappropriate erythropoietin production. Increased erythropoietin production in the absence of anemia or generalized hypoxia is due either to regional renal hypoxia or the ectopic production of erythropoietin by renal tumors. An increased erythropoietin level and/or erythropoietin in cystic fluid have been described in patients with a solitary renal cyst [101] multicystic disease [24] or polycystic kidney disease [61, 83]. The increased erythropoietin level has been explained as induced by the pressure of cystic formation and the impairment of microcirculation which causes local hypoxia of kidney tissue and stimulates erythropoietin production. Erythrocytosis and high serum erythropoietin levels has been reported for two patients on maintenance hemodialysis for glomerulonephritis and with acquired cystic disease [86]. The excessive erythropoietin secretion in the presence of erythrocytosis in these two patients is suggested to be either autonomous or stimulated by renal ischemia. Intrarenal circulation disturbed by cystic tumors may prevent the normal functioning of oxygen sensor in the kidney and disturb the normal feedback regulation of erythropoietin secretion. A similiar explanantion has been suggested for posttransplantation erythrocytosis associated with graft rejection or graft artery stenosis in patients who have undergone bilateral nephrectomy prior to transplantation [91]. The renal parenchymal diseases associated with erythrocytosis described by Basu und Stein [3], Sonneborn et al. [92] and Stack and Zabetakis [93] are of particular interest. For this posttransplant erythrocytosis the native kidneys were shown to have been responsible for the increased erythropoietin production. Here again it is evident that erythropoietin production by diseased kidney tissue escapes the physiological feedback regulation of erythropoietin production.

Ectopic production of erythropoietin by renal tumor cells causes erythrocytosis in patients [97] with renal cell carcinoma. Of 179 kidney tumors associated with erythrocytosis reviewed by Hammond and Winnick [43], 120 were hypernephromas, three Wilm's tumors and two sarcomas. The resolution of erythrocytosis after surgical removel of the tumor is direct proof that paraneoplastic erythrocytosis results from the inappropriate production of erythropoietin by tumor cells.

Acknowledgements. The authors wish to thank Mrs. Mirjana Jocić for help with the statistical aspects of the study, Mrs. Jovana Sušić for her secretarial assistance and Mrs. Karolina Udovički for her editing of the English text.

References

1. Anagnostou A, Kurtzman NA (1985) The anemia of chronic renal failure. Semin Nephrol 5: 115–127
2. Anagnostou A, Schade S, Barone J, Fried W (1977) Effects of partial hepatectomy on extrarenal erythropoietin production in rats. Blood 50: 457–462
3. Basu TK, Stein RM (1974) Erythrocytosis associated with chronic renal disease. Arch Intern Med 133: 442–447
4. Bischel MD, Neiman RS, Berne TV, Telfer N, Lukes RJ, Barbour BH (1972) Hypersplenism in the uremic hemodialyzed patient. Nephron 9: 146–161
5. Bozzini CE, De Voto FC, Tomino JM (1966) Decreased responsiveness of hematopoietic tissue to erythropoietin in acutely uremic rats. J Lab Clin Med 68: 411–417
6. Brown S, Caro J, Erslev AJ, Murray TG (1980) Spontaneous increase in erythropoietin and hematocrit values associated with transient liver enzyme abnormalities in an anephric patient undergoing hemodialysis. Am J Med 68: 280–284
7. Brunois JP, Lavaud S, Melin JP, Diebold M, Toupance O, Chanard J (1981) Acute hepatitis and eryhtropoiesis in chronically haemodialyzed patients. Nephron 28: 152–153
8. Caro J, Brown S, Miller O, Murray T, Erslev AJ (1979) Erythropoietin levels in uremic nephric and anephric patients. J Lab Clin Med 93: 449–458
9. Chandra M, Garcia JF, Miller ME, Waldbaum RS, Bluestone PA, McVicar M (1983) Normalization of hematocrit in a uremic patient receiving hemodialysis: role of erythropoietin. J Pediatr 103: 80–83
10. Chandra M, McVicar M, Clemons G (1986) Evidence of active inhibition of erythropoietin production in renal failure. Pediatr Res 20: 447A
11. Chandra M, McVicar M, Clemons G, Mossey RT, Wilkes BM (1987) Role of erythropoietin in the reversal of anemia of renal failure with continuous ambulatory peritoneal dialysis. Nephron 46: 312–315
12. Chandra M, Miller ME, Garcia JF, Mossey RT, McVicar M (1985) Serum immunoreactive erythropoietin levels in patients with polycystic kidney disease as compared with other hemodialysis patients. Nephron 39: 26–29
13. Cohen RA, Clemons G, Ebbe S (1985) Correlation between bioassay and radioimmunoassay for erythropoietin in human serum and urine concentrates. Proc Soc Exp Biol Med 179: 296–299
14. Coleman JC, Eastwood JB, Curtis JR, Fox RA (1972) Hepatitis and hepatitis associated antigen (EHAA) in haemodialysis unit with observations on hemoglobin levels. Br J Urol 44: 194–201
15. Cotes PM (1982) Immunoreactive erythropoietin in serum, I Evidence for the validity of the assay method and the physiological relevance of estimates. Br J Haematol 50: 427–438
16. Cotes PM, Brozovic B, Mansell M, Samsond DM (1980) Radioimmunoassay of erythropoietin (Ep) in human serum: validation and application of an assay system. Exp Hematol 8 [Suppl 8]: 292–294
17. Dagher FJ, Ramos E, Erslev AJ, Alongi SV, Carmi SA, Caro J (1979) Are the native kidneys responsible for erythrocytosis in renal allorecipients? Transplantation 28: 496–498
18. Danilović V (1979) Endemic nephropathy in Yugoslavia. In: Strahinjić S, Stefanović V (eds) Endemic (Balkan) nephropathy. Proceedings of the 4th Symposium on endemic (Balkan) nephropathy. Institute of Nephrology and Hemodialysis, University of Niš, Niš, pp 7–10
19. Danilović V, Djurišić M, Mokranjac M, Stojimirović B, Živojinović J, Stojaković P (1957) Nëphrites chroniques provoquees par l'intoxication au plomb par voie digestive (farine). Presse Med 65: 2039–2040
20. Davies S, Glynne-Jones E, Bisson M, Bisson P (1975) Plasma erythropoietin assay in patients with chronic renal failure. J Clin Pathol 28: 875–878
21. de Klerk G, Wilmink JM, Rosengarten PCJ, Vet RJWM, Goudsmit R (1982) Serum erythropoietin (ESF) titers in anemia of chronic renal failure. J Lab Clin Med 100: 720–734

22. Delwishe F, Segal GM, Eschbach JW, Adamson JW (1986) Hematopoietic inhibitors in chronic renal failure: lack of in vitro specificity. Kidney Int 29: 641–648
23. Djukanović Lj, Biljanović-Paunović L, Mimić-Oka J, Pavlović-Kentera V (1989) The effect of sera from hemodialysis patients on erythroid colony growth in vitro. Period Biol (in press)
24. Donati RM, McCarthy JM, Lange RD, Gallagher NI (1963) Erythrocythemia and neoplastic tumors. Ann Intern Med 58: 47–55
25. Egrie JC, Cotes PM, Lane J, Das REG, Tam RC (1987) Development of radioimmunoassays for human erythropoietin using recombinant erythropoietin as tracer and immunogen. J Immunol Methods 99: 235–241
26. Erslev AJ (1983) Anemia of chronic renal failure. In: Williams WJ, Beutler E, Erslev AJ, Lichtman MA (eds) Hematology, 3rd edn. McGraw-Hill, New York, pp 417–425
27. Eschbach JW, Adamson JW (1985) Anemia of end-stage renal disease (ESRD). Kidney Int 38: 1–5
28. Eschbach JW, Cook JD, Scribner BH, Finch CA (1977) Iron balance in hemodialysis patients. Ann Intern Med 87: 710–713
29. Eschbach JW, Egrie JC, Downing MR, Browne JK, Adamson JW (1987) Correction of the anemia of end-stage renal disease with recombinant human erythropoietin. Results of a combined phase I and II clinical trial. N Engl J Med 316: 73–78
30. Eschbach JW, Funk D, Adamson J, Kuhn I, Scribner BH, Finch CA (1967) Erythropoiesis in patients with renal failure undergoing chronic dialysis. N Engl J Med 276: 653–658
31. Fisher JW (1980) Mechanism of the anemia of chronic renal failure. Nephron 25: 106–111
32. Fisher JW, Hatch FE, Roh BL, Allen RC, Kelley BJ (1968) Erythropoietin inhibitor in kidney extracts and plasma from anemic human subjects. Blood 31: 440–452
33. Freedman MH, Cattran DC, Saunders EF (1983) Anemia of chronic renal failure: inhibition of erythropoiesis by uremic serum. Nephron 35: 15–19
34. Freedman MH, Grunberger T, Saunders EF (1982) Erythropoietin inhibitors in uremic serum. Clin Invest Med 5: 237–240
35. Freedman MH, Saunders EF, Cattran DC, Rabin EZ (1983) Ribonuclease inhibition of erythropoiesis in anemia of uremia. Am J Kidney Dis 2: 530–533
36. Fried W (1970) The liver as a source of extrarenal erythropoietin. Blood 40: 671–677
37. Fried W (1981) Hematologic abnormalities in chronic renal failure. Semin Nephrol 1: 176–187
38. Fürst P, Zimmerman L, Bergström J (1976) Determination of endogenous middle molecules in normal and uremic body fluids. Clin Nephrol 5: 178–188
39. Gallagher NI, McCarthy JM, Hart KT, Lange RD (1959) Evaluation of plasma erythropoietic stimulating factors in anemic uremic patient. Blood 14: 662–667
40. Garcia JF, Sherwood J, Goldwasser E (1979) Radioimmunoassay of erythropoietin. Blood Cells 5: 405–419
41. Goldsmith HJ, Ahmad R, Raichura N, Lal SM, McConnell CA, Gould DA, Gyde OHB, Green J (1982) Association between rising haemoglobin concentration and renal cyst formation in patients on long term regular haemodialysis treatment. Proc Eur Dial Transplant Assoc 19: 313–318
42. Gutman RA, Huang AT (1980) Inhibitor of marrow thymidine incorporation from sera of patients with uremia. Kidney Int 18: 715–724
43. Hammond D, Winnick S (1974) Paraneoplastic erythrocytosis and ectopic erythropoietins. Ann NY Acad Sci 230: 219–227
44. Hocking WG (1987) Hematologic abnormalities in patients with renal diseases. Hematol Oncol Clin North Am 1: 229–259
45. Joske RA, McAlister JM, Prankerd TAJ (1956) Isotope investigations of red cell production and destruction in chronic renal disease. Clin Sci 15: 511–522
46. Koch KM, Radtke HW (1979) Role of erythropoietin deficiency in the pathogenesis of renal anemia. Klin Wochenschr 57: 1031–1036
47. Kolk-Vegter AJ, Bosch E, VanLeeuven AM (1971) Influence of serum hepatitis on haemoglobin level in patients on regular hemodialysis. Lancet 1: 526–528

48. Kominami N, Lowrie EG, Ianhez LE, Skaren A, Hampers CL, Merrill JP, Lange RD (1971) The effect of total nephrectomy on hematopoiesis in patients undergoing chronic hemodialysis. J Lab Clin Med 78: 524–532
49. Lacombe C, Da Silca J-L, Bruneval P, Fournier J-G, Wendling F, Casadevall N, Camilleri J-P, Bariety J, Varet B, Tambourin P (1988) Peritubular cells are the site of erythropoietin synthesis in the murine hypoxic kidney. J Clin Invest 81: 620–623
50. Lamperi S, Carozzi S (1985) T lymphocytes, monocytes and eryhtropoiesis disorders in chronic renal failure. Nephron 39: 211–215
51. Lange RD, Gallagher NI (1962) Clinical and experimental observations on the relationship of the kidney of erythropoietin production. In: Jacobson LO, Doyle M (eds) Erythropoiesis. Grune and Stratton, New York, pp 361–373
52. Loge JP, Lange RD, Moore CV (1958) Characterization of the anemia associated with chronic renal insufficiency 24: 4–18
53. Markson JL, Rennie JB (1956) The anemia of chronic renal insufficiency: the effect of serum from azotaemic patients on maturation of normoblasts in suspension culture. Scott Med J 1: 320–322
54. McGonigle RJS, Boineau FG, Beckman B, Ohene-Frempong K, Lewy JE, Shadduck RK, Fisher JW (1985) Erythropoietin and inhibitors of in vitro erythropoiesis in the development of anemia in children with renal disease. J Lab Clin Med 105: 449–458
55. McGonigle RJS, Husserl F, Wallin JD, Fisher JW (1984) Hemodialysis and conitnuous ambulatory peritoneal dialysis effects on erythropoiesis in renal failure. Kidney Int 25: 430–436
56. McGonigle RJS, Wallin JD, Husserl F, Deftos LJ, Rice JC, O'Neill WJ Jr (1984) Potential role of parathyroid hormone as an inhibitor of erythropoiesis in the anemia of renal failure. J Lab Clin Med 104: 1016–1026
57. McGonigle RJS, Wallin JD, Shadduck RK, Fisher JW (1984) Erythropoietin deficiency and inhibition of erythropoiesis in renal insufficiency. Kidney Int 25: 437–444
58. Meyrier A, Simon P, Boffa G, Brissot P (1981) Uremia and the liver. I: The liver and erythropoiesis in chronic renal failure. Nephron 29: 3–6
59. Meytes D, Bogin E, Ma A, Dukes PP, Massry SG (1981) Effect of parathyroid hormone on erythropoiesis. J Clin Invest 67: 1263–1269
60. Mirand EA, Murphy GP (1971) Erythropoietin activity in anephric humans given prolonged androgen treatment. J Surg Oncol 3: 59
61. Mirand EA (1968) Extra-renal and renal control of eryhtropoietin production. Ann NY Acad Sci 149: 94–106
62. Mladenovic J, Eschbach JW, Garcia JF, Adamson JW (1984) The anemia of chronic renal failure in sheep: studies in vitro. Br J Haematol 58: 491–500
63. Moriyama Y, Saito H, Kinoshita Y (1970) Erythropoietin inhibitor in plasma from patients with chronic renal failure. Haematologia 4: 15–22
64. Morra L, Ponassi A, Gurreri G, Moccia F, Caristo G, Mela GS, Saccheti C (1987) Alterations of erythropoiesis in chronic uremic patients treated with intermittent hemodialysis. Biomed Pharmacother 41: 396–399
65. Muller-Wiefel DE, Schärer K (1983) Serum erythropoietin levels in children with chronic renal failure. Kidney Int 15: S70–S76
66. Naets JP, Garcia JF, Toussaint C, Buset M, Waks D (1986) Radioimmunoassay of erythropoietin in chronic uraemia or anephric patients. Scand J Haematol 37: 390–394
67. Naets JP, Heuse A (1962) Measurement of erythropoietic stimulating factor in anemic patients with or without renal disease. J Lab Clin Med 60: 365–374
68. Naets JP, Wittek M (1968) Erythropoiesis in anephric man. Lancet 2: 941–943
69. Najean Y, Vignerol N, Eberlin A, Dresch C, Delon S, Naret C, Petrover M, Aubert P (1983) L'anemie de l'insuffisance renale I Mecanismes de l'anemie des sujets traites par hemodialyse periodique. Presse Med 12: 1063–1066
70. Ohno Y, Rege AB, Fisher JW, Barone J (1978) Inhibitors of erythroid colony forming cells (CFU-E and BFU-E) in sera of azotemic patients with anemia of renal disease. J Lab Clin Med 92: 916–923

71. Ortega JA, Malekzadeh MH, Dukes PP, Andrew MA, Pennisi AV, Fine PN, Shore NA (1977) Exceptionally high serum erythropoietin activity in an anephric patient with severe anemia. Am J Hematol 2: 299–306
72. Ortega JA, Malekzadeh MH, Dukes PP, Pennisi AV, Fine RN, Ma A, Shore NA (1979) A beneficial effect of the in situ kidney on in vitro marrow erythropoiesis in chronic renal failure. Nephron 23: 169–173
73. Pavlović-Kentera V, Clemons GK, Djukanović Lj, Biljanović-Paunović L (1987) Erythropoietin and anemia in chronic renal failure. Exp Hematol 15: 785–789
74. Pavlović-Kentera V, Djukanović Lj, Biljanović-Paunović L, Stojanović N, Milenković P (1987) Inhibitors of erythropoiesis in patients with chronic renal failure. In: Najman A, Guigon M et al. (eds) The inhibitors of hematopoiesis. INSERM Libbey, London, pp 133–136
75. Pololi-Anagnostou L, Westenfelder C, Anagnostou A (1981) Marked improvement of erythropoiesis in an anephric patient. Nephron 29: 277–279
76. Radtke HW, Claussner A, Erbes PM, Scheuermann EH, Schoeppe W, Koch KM (1979) Serum erythropoietin concentration in chronic renal failure: relationship to degree of anemia and excretory renal function. Blood 54: 877–883
77. Radtke HW, Erbes PM, Fassbinder W, Koch KM (1977) The variable role of erythropoietin deficiency in the pathogenesis of dialysis anaemia. Proc Eur Dial Transplant Assoc Proc 14: 177–183
78. Radtke HW, Erbes PM, Schippers E, Koch KM (1978) Serum erythropoietin concentration in anephric patients. Nephron 22: 361–365
79. Radtke HW, Frei U, Erbes PM, Schoeppe W, Koch KM (1980) Improving anemia by hemodialysis: effect of serum erythropoietin. Kidney Int 17: 382–387
80. Radtke HW, Rege AB, LaMarche MD, Bartos D, Bartos F, Campbell RA, Fisher JW (1981) Identification of spermine as an inhibitor of erythropoiesis in patients with chronic renal failure. J Clin Invest 67: 1623–1629
81. Raich PC, Korst DR (1978) Plasma erythropoietin levels in patients undergoing long-term hemodialysis. Arch Pathol Lab Med 102: 73–75
82. Rege AB, Brookins J, Fisher JW (1982) A radioimmunoassay for erythropoietin: serum levels in normal human subjects and patients with hemopoietic disorders. J Lab Clin Med 100: 829–843
83. Rosse WF, Waldmann TA, Cohen P (1963) Renal cysts, erythropoietin and polycythemia. Am J Med 34: 76–81
84. Schuster SJ, Wilson JH, Erslev AJ, Caro J (1987) Physiologic regulation and tissue localization of renal erythropoietin messenger RNA. Blood 70: 316–318
85. Segal GM, Stueve T, Adamson JW (1987) Spermine and spermidine are non-specific inhibitors of in vitro hematopoiesis. Kidney Int 31: 72–76
86. Shalhoub RJ, Rajan U, Kim VV, Goldwasser E, Klark JA, Antoniou LD (1982) Erythrocytosis in patients on long-term hemodialysis. Ann Intern Med 97: 686–690
87. Shannon JS, Lappin TRJ, Elder GE, Roberts GM, McGeown MG, Bridges JM (1985) Increased plasma glycosidase and protease activity in uraemia: possible role in the aetiology of the anaemia of chronic renal failure. Clin Chim Acta 153: 203–207
88. Sherwood JB, Goldwasser E (1979) A radioimmunoassay for erythropoietin. Blood 54: 885–893
89. Sherwood JB, Charmichael LD, Goldwasser E (1988) The heterogeneity of circulating human serum erythropoietin. Endocrinology 122: 1472–1477
90. Simon P, Meyrier A, Tanquerel T, Ang KS (1980) Improvement of anaemia in haemodialysis pateints after viral or toxic hepatic cytolisis. Br Med J 280: 892–898
91. Sinnassamy P, O'Regan S (1987) Polycythemia in pediatric renal transplantation. Clin Nephrol 27: 242–244
92. Sonneborn R, Perez GO, Epstein M, Martelo O, Pardo V (1977) Erythrocytosis associated with the nephrotic syndrome. Arch Intern Med 137: 1068–1072
93. Stack JI, Zabetakis M (1979) Erythrocytosis associated with idiopathic membranous glomerulopathy. Clin Nephrol 12: 87–89

94. Stefanović S, Savin S, Pendić S, Ristić MM, Jančić MS, Pavlović-Kentera V, Banićević B, Veljović R, Glidžić L (1971) Pathogenie de l'anemie dans l'insuffisance renale chronique. Bordeaux Med 4: 821–826
95. Swartz R, Dombrouski J, Burnatowska-Hledin M, Mayor G (1987) Microcytic anemia in dialysis patients: reversible marker of aluminum toxicity. Am J Kidney Dis 9: 217–223
96. Thevenod F, Radtke HW, Grützmacher P, Vincent E, Koch K M, Schoeppe W, Fassbinder W (1983) Deficient feedback regulation of erythropoiesis in kidney transplant patients with polycythemia. Kidney Int 24: 227–232
97. Thorling EB (1972) Paraneoplastic erythrocytosis and inappropriate erythropoietin production. Scand J Haematol [Suppl 17]: 11–80
98. Tielemans C, Collart F, Wens R, Smeyers-Verbeeke J, van Hooff I, Dratwa M, Verbeelen D (1985) Improvement of anemia with deferoxamine in hemodialysis patients with aluminum-induced bone disease. Clin Nephrol 24: 237–241
99. Urabe A, Saito T, Fukamachi H, Kubota M, Takaku F (1987) Serum erythropoietin titers in the anemia of chronic renal failure and other hematological states. Int J Cell Cloning 5: 202–208
100. Van Dyke D, Keighley G, Lawrence J (1963) Decreased responsiveness to erythropoietin in a patient with anemia secondary to chronic uremia. Blood 22: 838–842
101. Vertel RM (1967) Solitary renal cyst. Arch Intern Med 120: 54
102. Walle AJ, Wong GY, Clemons GK, Garcia JF, Niedermayer W (1987) Erythropoietin-hematocrit feedback circuit in the anemia of end-stage renal disease. Kidney Int 31: 1205–1209
103. Wallner SF, Vautrin RM (1978) The anemia of chronic renal failure: studies of the effect of organic solvent extraction of serum. J Lab Clin Med 92: 363–369
104. Wallner SF, Vautrin RM (1981) Evidence that inhibition of erythropoiesis is important in the anemia of chronic renal failure. J Lab Clin Med 97: 170–178
105. Wallner SF, Vautrin RM, Kurnick JE, Ward HP (1978) The effect of serum from patients with chronic renal failure on erythroid colony growth in vitro. J Lab Clin Med 92: 370–375
106. Wallner SF, Ward HP, Vautrin R, Alfrey AC, Mishell J (1975) The anemia of chronic renal failure: in vitro response of bone marrow to erythropoietin. Proc Soc Exp Biol Med 149: 939–944
107. Winderoë TE, Sanengen T, Halvorsen S (1983) Erythropoietin and uremic toxicity during continuous ambulatory peritoneal dialysis. Kidney Int 24 [Suppl 16]: S208–S217
108. Winearls CG, Oliver DO, Pippard MJ, Reid C, Downing MR, Cotes PM (1986) Effect of human erythropoietin derived from recombinant DNA on the anemia of patients maintained by chronic haemodialysis. Lancet 2 (8517): 1175–1178
109. Winearls CG, Cotes PM, Pippard M, Reid C, Oliver DO (1987) Correction of anemia in haemodialysis patients with recombinant erythropoietin – follow up and results of pharmakokinetic, ferrokinetic and bone marrow culture studies. Abstract of the Xth International Congress on Nephrology, London, p 183
110. Yawata Y, Jacob HS (1975) Abnormal red cell metabolism in patients with chronic uremia: nature of the defect and its persistence despite adequate hemodialysis. Blood 45: 231–239
111. Zappacosta AR, Caro J, Erslev A (1982) Normalization of hematocrit in patients with end-stage renal disease on continuous ambulatory peritoneal dialysis. The role of erythropoietin. Am J Med 72: 53–57
112. Zaroulis CG, Hoffman BJ, Kourides IA (1981) Serum concentrations of erythropoietin measured by radioimmunoassay in hematologic disorders and chronic renal failure. Am J Hematol 11: 85–92
113. Zucker S, Lysik RM, Mohammed G (1976) Erythropoiesis in chronic renal disease. J Lab Clin Med 88: 528–535

Renal Artery Stenosis and Renal Polyglobulia

P. GRÜTZMACHER and W. SCHOEPPE

Clinical Characteristics and Mechanisms of Renal Polyglobulias

Renal polyglobulia is characterized by an excess secretion of erythropoietin by the kidney in the absence of systemic hypoxaemia. A decrease in blood oxygen tension is the principle signal for the production of erythropoietin. The sensor is undoubtedly located in the kidney, however, neither its excact site nor the site of the production and the secretion of erythropoietin are yet fully elucidated. There is growing evidence that renal erythropoietin is produced by peritubular interstitial cells of the outer medulla and the cortex [41], although cultured mesangial cells have been found able to produce the hormone as well [40]. In detail the regulation of the production of erythropoietin is handled elsewhere in this book (Pagel et al., this volume).

The mechanisms of the inadequate secretion of erythropoietin in renal polyglobulia are mainly attributed to either local hypoxia of kidney tissue or to proliferation of malignant cells. Polyglobulia has been observed in patients with several renal tumors, expecially hypernephromas, but also sarcomas, adenomas and some other extrarenal tumors [51]. Severe unilateral hydronephrosis can enhance the secretion of erythropoietin by the obstructed kidney in the presence of exhausting excretory function [37].

Polyglobulia may develop in a number of patients with polycystic kidney disease. However, the concomitant development of metabolic disturbances related to uraemia usually counteracts the manifestation of significant polycythaemia. In comparison with patients with other renal diseases at a similar stage of chronic renal insufficiency, the stimulated erythropoietin secretion is at least accompanied by a less severe anaemia. In patients with solitary renal cysts, development of polyglobulia has been observed occasionally. Although a high erythropoietin concentration is often found in the fluid of these cysts or in the cyst wall, secretion of erythropoietin into the systemic circulation is mostly insignificant [2, 3, 28, 37].

After kidney transplantation, erythrocytosis due to an excess secretion of erythropoietin develops in a portion of patients [1, 30, 33, 57]. In a series of 82 consecutive renal transplant recipients with well-functioning grafts we observed erythrocytosis in 12 patients of our unit [56]. Although renal anaemia has been present in these patients prior to transplantation, not the grafted but the native, frequently shrunken kidneys have been recognized as the source of excess erythropoietin by determination of erythropoietin levels in the renal veins. It is assumed that the shrinkage of the native kidneys induces tissue hypoxia, hereby stimulation erythropoietin secretion which is nonetheless limited and which can induce erythrocytosis only when the uraemic milieu is reversed by sufficient graft function. Frequently, these patients require intermittent phlebotomies to prevent thromboembolic complications. Nephrectomy of the native kidneys leads to the normalization of erythropoiesis and erythropoietin serum concentration [13].

Finally, polyglobulia has been reported in patients with renal artery stenosis, which has been presumed to be a typical condition for the induction of kidney hypoxia. This will be discussed in detail below.

Hypertension and Polyglobulia

Some polyglobulic syndromes are associated with renal hypertension: Simultaneous stimulation of both erythropoietin and the renin-angiotensin system is common in renal artery stenosis, polycystic kidney disease and post-transplant erythrocytosis. Patients with solitary renal cysts, unilateral hydronephrosis and renal tumors frequently present with normal blood pressure [3, 37].

In patients with endocrine hypertension secondary to pheochromocytomas, hyperthyroidism and Cushings disease, polycythaemia develops occasionally; the mechanisms are attributed to either renal vasoconstriction or an increased oxygen consumption stimulating the secretion of erythropoietin or to an additive erythropoietic activity of these hormones [17, 34, 37].

Mild to moderate hypertension may occur in patients with polycythaemia vera, originating from an increased peripheral resistance due to altered blood viscosity in accordance with the rule of Hagen-Pouseuille. Here, both renin and erythropoietin levels are regularly normal or decreased [12, 14, 16]. Secondary polyglobulia of pulmonary diseases is usually not associated with hypertension.

A diminished plasma volume resulting in pseudopolyglobulia has been observed in a small cohort of patients with essential hypertension [8, 52, 54]. It is assumed that these patients belong to the high-renin essential hypertension subgroup [55]. Besides the known effect of high-dose diuretic therapy, pseudopolyglobulia has been found in patients not on diuretic drugs and was attributed to an increased vascular tone effecting a shift of intravasal fluid to the interstitial space and an increased glomerular filtration [55]. In patients with a severe nephrotic syndrome pseudopolyglobulia develops more frequently [3].

Relationship Between the Regulation of Erythropoietin and Renin

Under various clinical and experimental conditions, it could be shown that the secretion of renin and erythropoietin can be regulated independently of one an other [34, 37]. However, many diseases alter the regulation of both hormones in a similar way. As shown by intravenous administration of the recombinant human derivative, erythropoietin has neither a direct effect on blood pressure [50], nor does it entail a release of renin (Gruetzmacher, unpublished observation). However, intravenous injection of renin increases the secretion of erythropoietin in the presence of hypoxaemia; under normal oxygen tension this effect is only minimal [25].

Angiotension II-induced vasoconstriction seems to aggravate tissue hypoxia under extremely low oxygen tension, hereby acting as an indirect stimulus for the secretion of erythropoietin [26]. On the other hand, hypoxaemia is a potent stimulus for the secretion of erythropoietin, while only a marginal effect on the secretion of renin can be observed [26, 34, 59].

It has been recognized in the meantime that the kidney produces and secrets erythropoietin in a biologically active form, as evidenced by the detection of messenger RNA of erythropoietin [41] and perfusion studies of isolated kidneys [7]. Earlier concepts supposed the kidney to secret (a) an enzyme, called erythrogenin, which activated a circulating, inactive prohormone synthesized by the liver [9, 23, 60, 61], or (b) an inactive erythropoetic precursor, which was activated by a circulating factor presumably produced by the liver [38, 39]. Although these theories can now be considered as clearly refuted, some effects of angiotensin II, renin and renin substrate have been interpreted as further support of the concept of the secretion of erythropoietin as a prohormone. In crude erythropoietin preparations certain reninlike activity has been reported [24]. However, the intravenous administration of the recombinant human erythropoietin did not show any effect on blood pressure and plasma renin levels.

Stimulation of the growth of erythropoetic precursor cells by a renin substrate and by angiotensin II has been observed [5, 21, 49]. Furthermore, some immunological cross reactions between erythropoietin and renin substrate have been observed by using antisera against erythropoietin [22]. Based on these and other findings, the hypothesis has been proposed that renin substrate could contain erythropoietin [21, 22]. Meanwhile, the amino acid sequences of both erythropoietin and angiotensinogen have been identified [32, 48]. As these turned out to be clearly different, this theory can no longer be maintained. Yet it remains unanswered, whether these intriguing similarities between the two hormonal systems can be evoked only because of technical difficulties, e.g. the use of antisera with low specificity or the use of crude tissue preparations containing both hormones.

Secretion of Erythropoietin and Erythropoesis in Renal Artery Stenosis

Experimental Investigations

It could be demonstrated in several animal studies that the concentration of erythropoietin in the renal vein increased after experimental constriction of the renal artery [11, 18, 19, 27, 45, 46, 49, 53]. However, this could not be confirmed by others [10, 44]. An increase of the urinary erythropoietin excretion as well as an increased erythropoietin concentration in kidney extracts was observed in rabbits after clamping of the renal artery [29]. Furthermore, torsion of the vascular pedicle increased also the erythropoietin concentration in the renal veins [43]. The observed increment of the erythropoietin concentration in the renal veins of stenotic kidneys was not always accompanied by changes of the systemic erythropoietin level, if measured at all. This suggests that the decrease in renal blood flow could be a reason for an increased serum concentration in the renal vein of a stenotic kidney in the presence of an unchanged secretion rate. Finally, enhanced erythropoesis has been observed only in some of the animals investigated [18, 29, 53].

Clinical Investigations

Up to now, clinical data on the effects of renal artery stenoses on the regulation of the secretion of erythropoietin and erythropoesis are rare. Cases of polyglobulia have been observed in patients with renal artery stenosis [6, 14, 20, 31, 42, 54]. In some cases, polyglobulia disappeared after surgical correction of the stenosis [31, 42].

In the largest population studied, described by Tarazi [54] and Frohlich [20], an elevated haematocrit was found in 33 of 148 patients with renovascular hypertension. However, no details about drug therapy, especially the amount of diuretics, were stated. Thus it might be assumed that diuretic treatment, which was one of the primary antihypertensive regimens in the 1960s, could have contributed to the high incidence of polyglobulia, which has not been observed by later investigators.

In a matched-pairs study, no difference in haematocrit and haemoglobin levels of patients with essential and renovascular hypertension could be demonstrated. However, only a small number of patients was included in this study [11].

Bourgoigne [6] found a slightly increased mean peripheral erythropoietin level in a group of 19 patients with renovascular hypertension in comparison with a control group of 14 patients with hypertension unrelated to renal disease. However, in all of four patients in whom renal vein determination of erythropoietin could be performed erythropoietin levels were normal in the renal veins and did not differ from the peripheral erythropoietin levels. Polyglobulia has not been observed in any of these patients either.

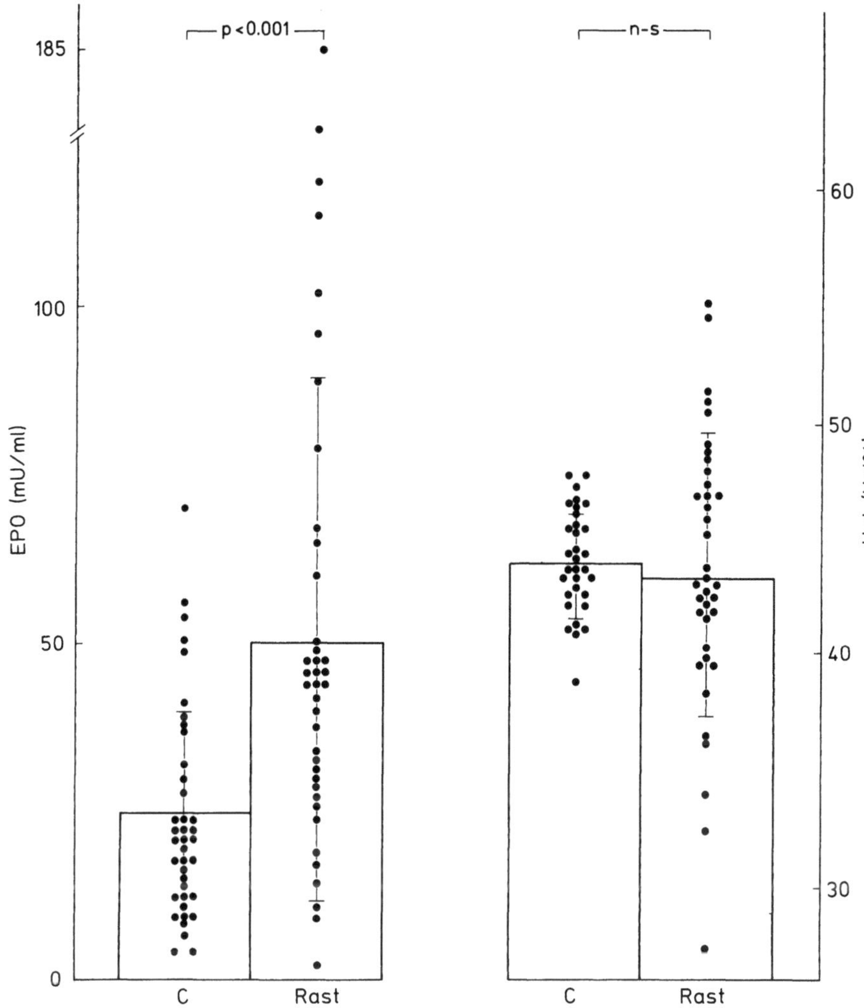

Fig. 1. Erythropoietin (*EPO*) level in peripheral venous blood and haematocrit (*Hct*) in patients with renal artery stenosis (*RAST*) and healthy controls (*C*), *n* = 37

Studies and Results

In our hospital, the prevalence of polyglobulia was studied in a consecutive series of 66 hypertensive patients with angiographically proven renal artery stenoses of different degrees. In all of these, diuretic treatment was discontinued for 5–7 days. Erythropoietin concentration was measured in 37 of these simultanously in peripheral and renal venous blood using the fetal mouse liver cell assay, i.e. a highly sensitive in vitro bio-assay [58]. The sensitivity limit of this assay was 2.5 mU/ml

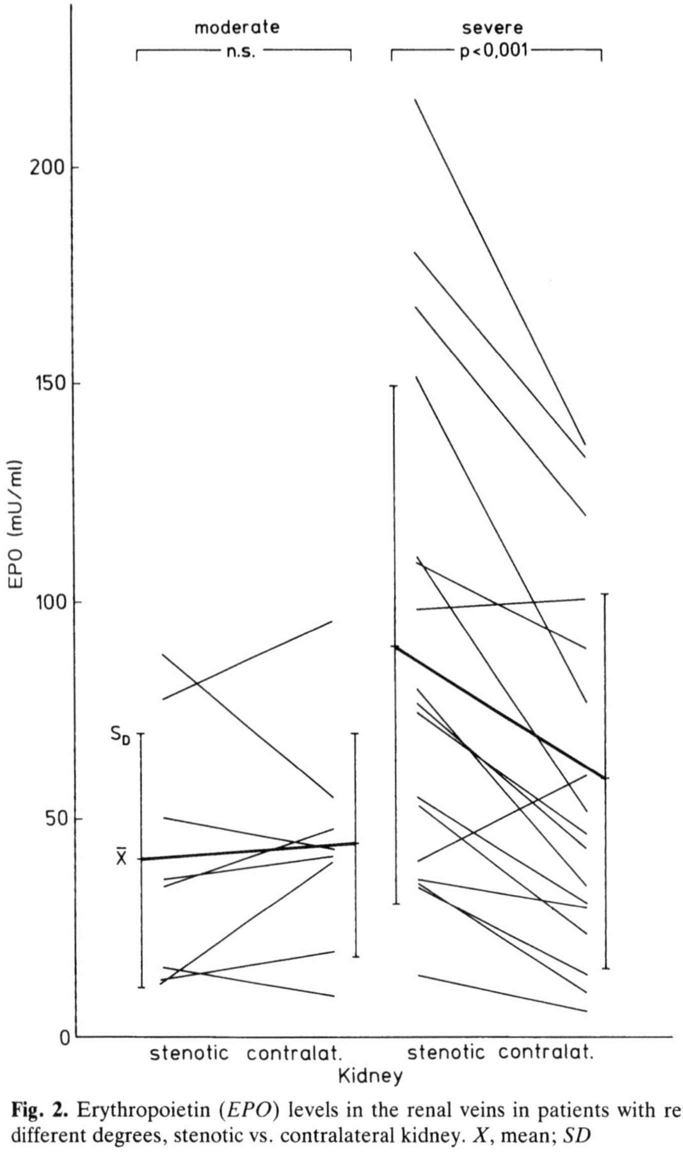

Fig. 2. Erythropoietin (*EPO*) levels in the renal veins in patients with renal artery stenoses of different degrees, stenotic vs. contralateral kidney. *X*, mean; *SD*

in our laboratory; technical details of this assay as well as several modifications have already been described [56]. As the peripheral venous erythropoietin level is identical to the arterial level, simultaneous measurement allows the estimation of arteriovenous differences.

The mean peripheral erythropoietin level in patients with renal artery stenosis was significantly higher than in a healthy and normotensive control group (Fig. 1).

Table 1. Comparison of mean haematocrit, haemoglobin concentration and erythrocyte counts in patients with renal artery stenoses and healthy controls

	Renal artery stenosis		Healthy controls	
n	Male 34	Female 32	Male 18	Female 18
Haematocrit (vol. %)	44.2 ± 5.7	41.3 ± 4.7	45.0 ± 1.7	43.1 ± 2.3
Haemoglobin (g/l)	149.0 ± 20	140 ± 15	148 ± 11	145 ± 9
Erythrocyte counts (10^{12}/l)	4.8 ± 0.6	4.6 ± 0.5	4.9 ± 0.4	4.6 ± 0.4

However, in most patients the erythropoietin levels were still in the normal range of 4–40 mU/ml. The mean peripheral erythropoietin level increased with increasing severity of the stenosis: In patients with a moderate stenosis, i.e. below 50%, the mean erythropoietin level of 35 ± 23 mU/ml (mean ± SD) was not significantly different from that of controls, while in patients with a severe stenosis, i.e. more than 50%, the mean erythropoietin level was markedly elevated to 64 ± 45 mU/ml ($P < 0.001$).

Measurement of erythropoietin in both renal veins yielded almost equal concentrations in patients with unilateral moderate stenosis. The mean erythropoietin concentration in the renal veins was only slightly above the mean peripheral venous level, resulting in a mean arteriovenous difference of less than 20%. In patients with severe stenoses, a considerable difference between the erythropoietin levels of both renal veins was found. The mean arteriovenous difference usually amounted to 40%–50% in the stenotic kidney, whereas the mean erythropoietin level in the contralateral renal vein was equal to the mean peripheral level, suggesting suppressed erythropoietin secretion by the contralateral kidney (Fig. 2). In six patients with bilateral stenoses, the mean peripheral erythropoietin level showed a slight and insignificant elevation to 33 ± 18 mU/ml. The mean erythropoietin levels were nearly equal in both renal veins when the side of major stenosis was compared with the less stenotic side.

Elevated haematocrit values were observed 6 of the 66 patients, however, in all of these, the increment was moderate, as Fig. 1 shows. The two males presented with 55% haematocrit, corresponding haemoglobin levels were 186 and 176 g/l; erythrocyte counts were 5.6 and 6.0 mU/ml. Both patients had moderate unilateral stenoses and normal erythropoietin levels of 10 and 18 mU/ml, respectively. The four females presented with haematocrits in the range of 46.5%–50.0%. Also in these patients haemoglobin levels and erythrocyte counts were in the borderline range. The erythropoietin concentration was slightly elevated to 60 mU/ml in one woman with a bilateral stenosis and was not measured in the other three women who exhibited severe unilateral stenoses.

The mean levels of haematocrit, haemoglobin and erythrocyte counts showed no differences between the whole patients group and healthy controls when compared according to sex (Table 1), but varied considerably more in patients with renal artery stenosis (Fig. 1). Furthermore, there was no significant difference between patients with moderate and severe unilateral or bilateral stenosis as well as complete occlusion.

Summary and Conclusion

As derived from experimental as well as clinical investigations, renal artery stenosis can increase the secretion of erythropoietin. However, comparing only side differences in renal veins, the amount of this stimulation is by far overestimated and may be mimiced by a concentrating effect of the reduced renal blood flow. So, a considerable number of patients probably has a normal renal erythropoietin secretion rate. In agreement with this is the finding that the peripheral erythropoietin concentration is normal in the majority of these patients. Compared with levels of healthy controls, however, the mean erythropoietin concentration of patients with renal artery stenosis as a whole group is distinctly higher. Furthermore, elevated systemic erythropoietin concentrations have been found in our as well as in other investigations. However, the concentrations in these patients, too, were markedly lower compared for instance with those in patients with posytransplant erythrocytosis [56] and patients with anaemia [7, 14].

Clinical and experimental data render clear evidence that polyglobulia may develop as a consequence of renal artery constriction. However, the information about the prevalence of polyglobulia in patients with renal artery stenosis is rare and in part contradictory. The high prevalence of 23 % observed by Tarazi [54] could not be confirmed in our study, in which the prevalence was only 10%. Moreover, in two other studies, comprising smaller numbers of patients, no patient presented with polyglobulia [6, 11]. The opposite effects on plasma volume of different antihypertensive strategies, using primarily either diuretics or vasodilating agents, should be considered when interpreting these data.

The borderline character of polycythaemia found in our study seems to be in accordance with the moderate elevation of erythropoietin serum concentration. However, polycythaemia was not always accompanied by elevated erythropoietin serum levels and vice versa in our study or in others [6].

Compared to the effects of anaemia, the stimulation of erythropoietin by renal artery constriction is markedly lower. Two main reasons have to be considered: Firstly, renal artery perfusion can be maintained normal if at least 30% of the artery is still patent; therefore tissue hypoxia will develop very late in these kidneys. Secondly, a reduction of oxygen supply may be compensated to a great extent by lower tubular sodium absorption when renal blood flow and glomerular filtration rate begins to decline. On the other hand, if severe tissue hypoxia develops, which can not be compensated for, the capacity for the secretion of erythropoietin may decrease as a consequence of a decreased metabolic potential or progressive tissue necrosis [47].

References

1. Bacon BR, Rothman SA, Ricanati ES, Rashad FA (1980) Renal artery stenosis with erythrocytosis after renal transplantation. Arch Intern Med 140: 1206–1211
2. Balcerzak SP, Bromberg PA (1975) Secondary polycythemia, Semin Hematol 12: 353–382
3. Basu TK, Stein RM (1974) Erythrocytosis associated with chronic renal disease. Arch Intern Med 133: 442–447
4. Berlin NI (1975) Diagnosis and classification of the polycythemias. Semin Hemat 12: 339–351
5. Bilsel YC, Wood EJ, Lange RD (1963) Angiotensin II and erythropoiesis. Proc Soc Exp Biol Med 114: 475–479
6. Bourgoignie JJ, Gallagher NI, Perry HM Jr., Kurz L, Warnecke MA, Donati RM (1968) Renin and erythropoietin in normotensive and in hypertensive patients. J Lab Clin Med 71: 523–536
7. Caro J, Schuster S, Besarab A, Erslev AJ (1986) Renal biogenesis of erythropoietin In: J.N. Rich: Molecular and Cellular Aspects of Erythropoietin and Erythropoiesis NATO ASI Series H, Cell Biology 8 (1987) 329–336
8. Chrysant SG, Frohlich ED, Adamopoulos PN, Stein PD, Whitcomb WH, Allen EW, Neller G (1976) Pathophysiologic significance of "stress" or relative polycythemia in essential hypertension, Am J Cardiol 37: 1069
9. Contrera JG, Gorden AS, Weintraub AH (1966) Extraction of an erythropoietin producing factor from a particulate fraction of rat kidney. Blood 28: 330–343
10. Cooper GW, Nocenti MR (1961) Unilateral renal ischaemia and erythropoietin. Proc Soc Exp Biol Med 108: 546–549
11. Cotes PM, Lowe RD (1963) The influence of renal ischaemia on red-cell formation. In: Wiliams PC (ed) Hormones and the kidneys. Academic, London, pp 187–194
12. Cotes PM, Doré CJ, Liu Yin JA, Lewis SM, Messinezy M, Pearson TC, Reid C (1986) Determination of serum immunoreactive erythropoietin in the investigation of erythrocytosis. N Engl J Med 315: 283–287
13. Dagher FJ, Ramos E, Erslev AJ, Alongi SV, Karmi SA, Caro J (1979) Are the native kidneys responsible for erythrocytosis in renal allografts? Transplantation 28: 496–498
14. De Klerk G, Rosengarten PCJ, Vet RJWM, Goudsmit R (1981) Serum erythropoietin (ESF) titers in anemia. Blood 58: 1164–1170
15. De Klerk G, Rosengarten PCJ, Vet RJWM, Goudsmit R (1981) Serum erythropoietin (ESF) titers in polycythemia. Blood 58: 1171–1174
16. Erslev AJ, Caro J (1983) Pathophysiology of erythropoietin. In: Dunn CDR (ed) Current concepts in erythropoiesis. Wiley, New York, pp 1–20
17. Essers U, Mühlhoff G, Rahn KH, Ochs G (1977) Erhöhte Erythropoietin-Sekretion bei Phäochromozytom. Med Welt 28: 877–881
18. Fisher JW, Schofield R, Porteous DD (1965) Effects of renal hypoxia on erythropoietin production. Br J Haematol 11: 382–388
19. Fisher JW, Samuels AI, Langston JW (1967) Effects of angiotensin and renal artery constriction on erythropoietin production. J Pharmacol Exp Ther 157: 618–625
20. Frohlich ED, Tarazi RD (1968) High hematocrit in hypertension and its relationship with renal arterial disease. Ann NY Acad Sci 149: 569–569
21. Fyhrquist R, Rosenlöf K, Grönhagen-Riska C, Hortling L, Tikkanen I (1984) Is renin substrate an erythropoietin precursor? Nature 308: 649–652
22. Fyhrquist F, Rosenlöf K, Grönhagen-Riska C, Räsänen V (1986) Renin substrate (angiotensinogen) as a possible erythropoietin precursor. Contrib Nephrol 50: 167–174
23. Gordon AS, Kaplan SM (1978) Erythrogenin (REF) In: Fisher JW (ed) Kidney hormones: Erythropoietin, vol 2. Academic, London, pp 187–230
24. Gould AB, Keighley G, Lowy PH (1968) On the presence of a renin-like activity in erythropoietin preparations. Lab Invest 18: 2–7

25. Gould AB, Goodman SA, Green D (1973) An in vivo effect of renin on erythropoietin formation. Lab Invest 28: 719–722
26. Gould AB, Goodman S, DeWolf R, Onesti G, Swartz C (1980) Interrelation of the renin system and erythropoietin in rats. J Lab Clin Med 96: 523–533
27. Gross DM, Mujovic VM, Jubiz W, Fisher JW (1976) Enhanced erythropoietin and prostaglandin E production in the dog following renal artery constriction. Proc Soc Exp Biol Med 151: 498–510
28. Gurney CW (1970) Polycythemias and anemias associated with renal diseases. In: Fisher JW (ed) Kidney hormones. Academic, London, pp 307–409
29. Hansen P (1964) Demonstration of erythropoietin in urine and in kidney extracts from rabbits with experimental constriction of the left renal artery. Acta Pathol Microbiol Scand 61: 514–520
30. Herforth A, Binswanger U, Largiader F, Frick P (1979) Hohe Hämoglobinkonzentration und hoher Hämatokrit bei Trägern von Nierenallotransplantaten. Schweiz Med Wochenschr 109: 1293–1298
31. Hudgson P, Pearce JMS, Yeates WK (1967) Renal artery stenosis with hypertension and high hematocrit. Br Med J 1: 18–21
32. Jacobs K, Shoemaker C, Rudersdorf R, et al. (1985) Isolation and characterization of genomic and cDNA clones of human erythropoietin. Nature 313: 806–810
33. Ianhez LE, Da Fonseca JA, Chocair PR, Maspes V, Sabbage E (1977) Polycythemia after kidney transplantation. Influence of the native kidneys on the production of hemoglobin. Urol Int 32: 382–392
34. Jelkmann W (1986) Renal erythropoietin: properties and production. Rev Physiol Biochem Pharmacol 104: 139–215
35. Jelkmann W, Bauer C (1981) Demonstration of high levels of erythropoietin in rat kidneys following hypoxic hypoxia. Pflugers Arch 392: 34–39
36. Kramer K, Deetje P (1960) Beziehungen des O_2-Verbrauchs der Niere zu Durchblutung und Glomerulusfiltrat bei Änderung des arteriellen Druckes. Pflugers Arch 271: 782–796
37. Krantz SB, Jacobson LO (1970) Erythropoietin and the regulation of erythropoiesis. University of Chicago Press, Chicago
38. Kuratowska Z (1968) The renal mechanism of the formation and inactivation of erythropoietin. Ann NY Acad Sci 149: 128–134
39. Kuratowska Z, Lewartowski B, Liponski B (1964) Chemical and biologic properties of an erythropoietic generating substance obtained from perfusates of isolated anoxic kidneys. J Lab Clin Med 64: 226–237
40. Kurtz A, Jelkmann W, Pfeilschifter J, Bauer C (1986) Erythropoietin production in cultures of rat renal mesangial cells. Contrib Nephrol 50: 175–187
41. Lacombe C, Da Silva JL, Bruneval P, Camilleri JP, Bariety J, Tambourin P, Varet B (1988) Identification of tissues and cells producing erythropoietin in the anemic mouse. Contrib Nephrol 66: 17–24
42. Luke RG, Kennedy AC, Stirling WB, McDonald GA (1965) Renal artery stenosis, hypertension and polycythemia. Br Med J 1: 164–166
43. Mantz JM, Cholevas M, Warter J (1960) Etudes sur l'hémopoiétine chez le rat blanc. II. Arguments en faveur de son origine rénale. C R Soc Biol 154: 1068–1071
44. Mitus WJ, Galbraith P, Gollekeri M, Toyama K (1964) Experimental renal erythrocytosis. I. Effects of pressure and vascular interference. Blood 24: 343–355
45. Mujovic VM, Fisher JW (1974) Effects of indomethacin on erythropoietin production in dogs following renal artery constriction. I. The possible role of prostaglandins in the generation of erythropoietin by the kidney. J Pharmacol Exp Ther 191: 575–580
46. Murphy GP, Mirand EA, Johnston GS, Schirmer HKA (1966) Erythropoietin release in hypertensive dogs with renal artery stenosis. Surg Forum 17: 499–500
47. Murphy GP, Mirand EA, Johnston GS, Schirmer HKA (1967) Correlation of renal metabolism with erythropoietin release in hypertensive dogs with renal artery stenosis. Invest Urol 4: 372–377

48. Nakanishi (1983) cited in Fyhrquist F, Rosenlöf K, Grönhagen-Riska C, Räsänen V (1986) Renin substrate (angiotensiogen) as a possible erythropoietin-precursor. Contrib Nephrol 50: 173
49. Nakao K, Shirakura T, Azuma M, Maekawa T (1967) Studies on erythropoietic action of angiotensin II. Blood 29: 754–760
50. Samtleben W, Baldamus CA, Bommer J, Fassbinder W, Nonnast-Daniel B, Gurland HJ (1988) Blood pressure changes during treatment with recombinant human erythropoietin. Contrib Nephrol 66: 114–122
51. Sherwood JB (1984) The chemistry and physiology of erythropoietin. Vitam Horm 41: 196–199
52. Stefanini M, Urbas JV, Urbas JE (1978) Gaisböck's syndrome: its hematologic, biochemical and hormonal parameters. Angiology 29: 520
53. Takaku F, Hirashima K, Nakao K (1962) Studies on the mechanism of erythropoietin production. I. Effect of unilateral constriction of the renal artery. J Lab Clin Med 59: 815–820
54. Tarazi RC, Frohlich ED, Dustan HP, Gifford RW Jr., Page HI (1966) Hypertension and high hematocrit. Another clue to renal arterial disease. Am J Cardiol 18: 855–858
55. Tarazi RC, Dustan HP, Frohlich ED, Gifford RW jr, Hoffman GC (1970) Plasma volume and chronic hypertension. Arch Intern Med 125: 835
56. Thevenod F, Radtke HW, Grützmacher P, Vincent E, Koch KM, Schoeppe W, Fassbinder W (1983) Deficient feedback regulation of erythropoesis in kidney transplant patients with polycythemia. Kidney Int 24: 227–232
57. Varkarakis MJ, Sampson D, Gerbas JR, Bender MA, Mirand EA, Murphy GP (1971) Polycythemia following renal transplantation unrelated to the allograft. J Surg Oncol 3: 157–161
58. Wardle DFH, Baker I, Malpas JS, Brighley PFM (1973) Bioassay for erythropoietin using fetal mouse liver cells. Br J Haematol 24: 49–56
59. Weimann DN, Williamson HE (1981) Hypoxemia increases renin secretion rate in anesthetized newborn lambs. Life Sci 29: 1887–1893
60. Wong KK, Zanjani ED, Cooper CW, Gordon AS (1968) The renal erythropoietic factor. I. Studies on its purification. Proc Soc Exp Biol Med 128: 67–70
61. Zanjani ED, McLauring WD, Gordon AS, Rappaport WA, Biggs JM, Gidari AS (1971) Biogenesis of erythropoietin: role of substrate for erythrogenin. J Lab Clin Med 77: 751–758

Erythrocytosis in Renal Graft Recipients

F. Stockenhuber, K. Geissler, W. Hinterberger, and P. Balcke

Anemia develops during the course of chronic renal failure with deterioration of excretory kidney function [1–3]. Erythropoietin (EPO) deficiency [1, 2] and uremic bone marrow intoxication [4, 5] have been implicated as major causative factors for the development of renal anemia. This concept is supported by the observation that shortly after kidney transplantation, and in the presence of good kidney function, most if not all transplant patients overcome their anemic state; their hematocrits once again begin to build up to become normal or close to normal [6, 7]. However, in some patients the hematocrit continues to rise even after complete correction of anemia, resulting in post-transplant erythrocytosis (PTE) [6–9].

Since differentiation and maturation of red cells is under the control of EPO, elevated EPO concentrations have been suspected as being responsible for the increased erythropoiesis in PTE patients [6–10]. Several pathogenetic factors have been implicated in the development of renal hypoxia resulting in elevated EPO levels, including cardiac insufficiency, pulmonary diseases, renal artery stenosis, rejection episodes, and cyclosporine nephrotoxicity [6, 9, 11, 12]. However, none of these conditions occurs more often in patients with PTE than in transplant patients with normal hematocrits [6, 8, 9, 12], thus excluding hypoxia as the cause of erythrocytosis. Recently, elevated peripheral EPO concentrations have been reported in patients with PTE [7, 13]. The authors claim that the native kidneys are the source of increased EPO production, contradicting the generally accepted concept that the damaged kidneys are unable to produce sufficient EPO in endstage renal failure [1, 2, 12, 14].

To elucidate further the regulation of erythropoiesis and the role of EPO in kidney transplant patients, we determined peripheral EPO concentrations and circulating stem cells in a group of patients with PTE and compared them to a similar group of patients with normal hematocrit.

Materials and Methods

Patients

Out of 137 patients with well-functioning kidney grafts, 12 patients (8.7%) developed a rapid increase in hematocrit from a mean of 23% to 55% within 7 months after transplantation. These patients represented one of the two groups studied. To prevent thromboembolic events in these patients the hematocrit was kept at around 55% by intermittent phlebotomy. With the removal of an average amount of 2000 ml blood (4 x 500 ml), the hematocrit ranged from 52% to 57% (PTE patients). Blood samples for EPO determination were obtained at least 3 weeks after the last phlebotomy. For comparison, from the kidney graft recipients with normal or slightly decreased hemotocrit, who never had phlebotomy, a second group of 12 patients was selected and designated "non-PTE patients" (hematocrit 34% to 41%). Although exact matching of the two groups was not possible, the group of non-PTE patients was selected as close as possible to the group of PTE patients with regard to underlying diagnosis, age, sex, duration of hemodialysis before transplantation, time between transplantation and present investigation, average hematocrit while on hemodialysis, arterial oxygen saturation, and serum creatinine concentration, as well as immunosuppressive therapy with cyclosporine and low-dose prednisolone. In both groups, cyclosporine blood trough levels were kept at 400 ng/ml (RIA method). Mean prednisolone dose was 7.5 mg per day.

Assay for EPO

A modification of the radioimmunoassay recently described by Eckardt et al. [15] was used for EPO determination. Phosphate buffered saline (PBS), pH 7.5, containing 0.1% bovine serum albumin (BSA) was used as diluent buffer for all reagents. All incubations were carried out at 4° C.

Test Procedure. Aliquots of the following were combined in Eppendorf reaction cups: (a) 100 μl of serum, or standard solutions (10–1100 mU EPO/ml), (b) 100 μl of diluted EPO antiserum (1:15 000), and (c) 20 μl of 30% BSA in PBS. After preincubation for 24 h, 100 μl of radiolabelled EPO (8×10^{-15} mol) was added and tubes were incubated for another 24 h. After the incubation, separation of bound vs free ligand was accomplished using a secondary antibody technique. For this purpose 100 μl (1 unit) of goat anti-rabbit gammaglobulin (Calbiochem) and 100 μl rabbit gammaglobulin (0.03 mg; Calbiochem) were added to the Eppendorf reaction cups to precipitate bound ligand. After incubation for 4 h the tubes were centrifuged at 9500 *g* for 30 min. The supernatant was aspirated and the pellet counted for ^{125}I radioactivity. Data were expressed as percent of binding in the absence of unlabelled EPO.

Quality Controls. The maximum amount of antibody-precipitable ^{125}I-EPO (as determined using 100 μl of diluent buffer instead of EPO standard) was approximately 52% of the total radioactivity added. Nonspecific binding (as determined using 100 μl of diluent buffer instead of antiserum) was about 1.5% of the total radioactivity added. The intraassay coefficient of variation (assessed by tenfold determination of a diluted serum sample with a mean of 58 mU/ml) was 2.2%. The interassay coefficient of variation of 10 assays was 9.5% for samples containing a mean of 50 mU recombinant human EPO. Estimates are expressed in international units (U) or milliunits per ml (mU/ml), i.e. 1000 miU equals 1 U, using as standard the second international reference preparation for erythropoietin.

Peripheral Stem Cell Assay

Cell Separation. Twenty millilitres of peripheral blood was collected in 4 ml EDTA under sterile conditions. Mononuclear cells were harvested after a Ficoll-Hypaque gradient centrifugation (400 g, 40 min, 1077 g/ml).

In Vitro Assay. Pluripotent (CFU-GEMM) as well as committed progenitor cells (BFU-E, CFU-GM) were assayed using a modification of the clonal assay described by Fauser and Messner [16]. Each plate contained 0.9% methylcellulose, 30% fetal calf serum, 10% BSA (Behring), 1 U/ml erythropoietin (Toyobo), alpha-thioglycerol (10 mol/l), 5% phytohem-agglutinin-leucocyte-conditioned medium and Iscove's modified Dulbecco's medium (Gibco). Peripheral blood mononuclear cells were plated in quadruplicate at 2.5 x 10^5 per ml. After a culture period of 14 days (37°, 5% CO_2 full humidity) cultures were examined under an inverted microscope. Aggregates with a least 40 translucent, dispersed cells were counted as CFU-GM. Bursts containing more than 100 red coloured cells were scored as BFU-E. CFU-GEMM were identified by their heterogeneous composition of translucent and hemoglobinized cells. Individual colonies suspected as CFU-GEMM were picked, transferred to glass an stained by May-Gruenwald-Giemsa for cytological examination under a light microscope. The clonal nature of mixed colonies was confirmed by the linear relationship between the numbers of colonies. The number of colonies of all types was determined and the number per 1 ml of blood was calculated based on the leucocyte count, the percentage of mononuclear cells in the blood, and the percentage of mononuclear cells in the population of cells obtained by Ficoll-Hypaque gradient centrifugation.

The measurements of cyclosporine blood levels were done by a radioimmunoassay (Sandimmun RIA Kit). In each case, trough levels were measured.

HLA Typing

HLA typing was done using a standard method according to the NIH [17].

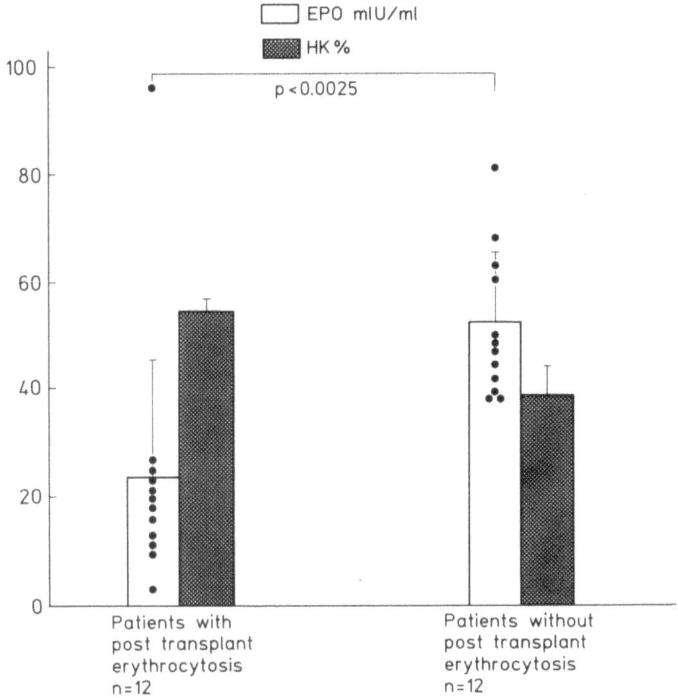

Fig. 1. Mean EPO concentration and hematocrit (HK) in 12 patients with PTE and 12 patients without PTE

Statistics

To evaluate the clinical data, we used Student's unpaired t test and comparison of binomial distribution.

Results

Figure 1 shows the mean EPO concentration and hematocrit in 12 patients with PTE and 12 patients without PTE. The mean serum EPO in PTE patients of 24 ± 23 (SD) miU/ml is significantly lower than the mean serum EPO of 53 ± 14 miU/ml in non-PTE patients ($p < 0.0025$).

Assaying peripheral stem cells reveals a significantly elevated BFU-E formation in PTE patients of 1230 ± 210 cells/ml as compared to BFU-E formation in non-PTE patients of 430 + 195 cells/ml ($p < 0.01$) (Fig. 2). In both groups CFU-GEMM and CFU-GM formation were within the normal range and showed no significant difference (data not shown).

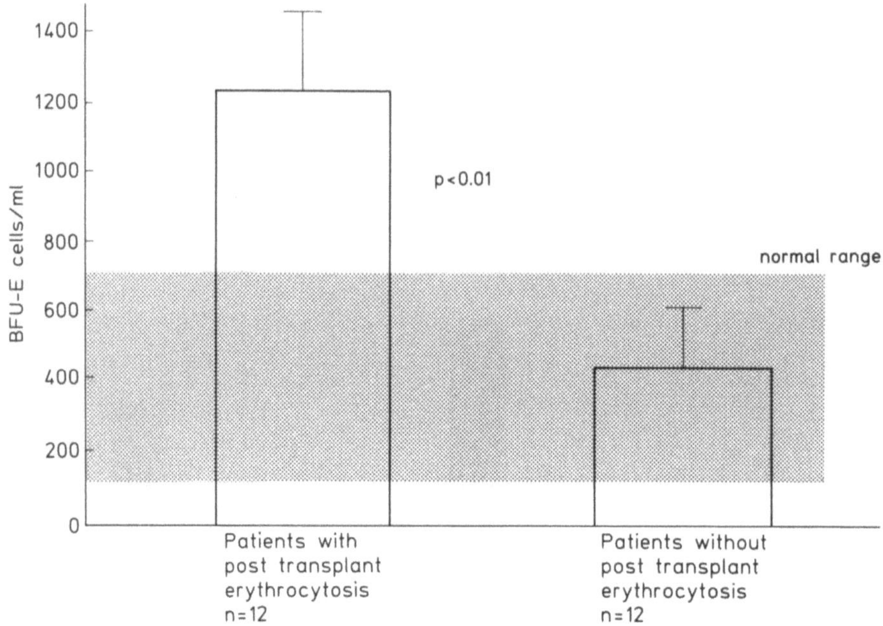

Fig. 2. BFU-E formation in 12 patients with PTE and 12 patients without PTE

HLA typing revealed a significantly increased incidence of the HLA-A_2 locus in our 12 PTE patients as compared to the non-PTE patients (10 out of 12 patients with PTE = 83% versus 53 out of 125 non-PTE patients = 42%, $p < 0.05$).

Discussion

After successful kidney transplantation renal function returns to normal. Therefore, it is not surprising that uremia-associated disturbances such as renal anemia usually disappear several months after transplantation. However, no convincing explanation has been offered so far for the consistent observation that in a certain percentage of transplant patients improvement of anemia progresses more rapidly and that production of erythrocytes continues after complete correction of the originally decreased red cell mass [8–10]. In general, the cause of the resulting polycythemia can be attributed to three different mechanisms. First, there may be autonomous red cell production as seen in patients suffering from polycythemia vera. Secondly, red cell production may rise to increase the oxygen transport when oxygenation is impaired, as in cardiopulmonary deseases or when kidney oxygenation is reduced due to severe renal artery stenosis [12], or as a consequence of kidney infarction [18–20]. And, thirdly, EPO production is increased without underlying hypoxia, as can be seen in some patients with hypernephroma, cerebellar carcinoma, or paraneoplastic syndrome [21].

Whereas the last two possibilities are associated with increased serum EPO concentrations, the first one is characterized by decreased serum EPO levels [22, 23]. In view of our evaluations of significantly decreased EPO levels in all but one patient with PTE and of the findings of Lamperi et al. [24], the possibility of autonomous red cell production seems to be most likely. Pulmonary disorders were excluded in every PTE patient by normal blood gases with arterial oxygen saturation of above 95%. Our results demonstrate that in most cases erythrocytosis is not induced by erythropoietin release from the kidney graft or the native kidneys. On the contrary, a feedbackdependent decrease of EPO serum levels was observed in patients with PTE, suggesting a restored normal intrarenal secretion [25]. Our findings appear connected to a higher development capacity of erythroid progenitors in the erythrocytotic patients that, in fact, can be due to early augmentation of EPO receptors on the cellular surface and consequently greater EPO sensitivity [26]. Such a particular sensitivity appears to be associated with the presence of the adherent mononuclear cell fraction and/or T lymphocytes in the medium. The removal of these cells is followed by a reduction in the number of BFU-E colonies per plate. Recently, various in vitro studies have been published [27, 28] which suggest that cyclosporine is able to increase the growth efficacy of bone marrow stem cells in the presence of T cells, possibly by inhibiting an endogenous, T cell-mediated suppressor mechanism. However, in our investigation no relationship could be found between the cyclosporine concentration and the development of eryhtrocytosis. In the one patient with PTE and elevated serum EPO, erythrocytosis seems to be due to increased EPO production without underlying hypoxia. Some authors [7, 13] assume this to be the case in most cases of PTE, using ex vivo, in vitro assays or bioassays for EPO determination. An interference of other growth factors, probably released from T cells, might be responsible for the differing results obtained by immunological EPO determination methods [24, 29].

Wondering whether a genetic predisposition could be involved, we investigated the HLA types by standard methods [17] in all patients. We found a high, significant prevalence of the HLA-A_2 locus in our patients with erythrocytosis, suggesting a HLA-associated genetic factor. The one patient with PTE and elevated EPO concentration did not have the HLA-A_2 locus.

The clinical conclusion of our study should be the following: Before one removes the native kidneys of patients with PTE, suspecting them as an effusive source of EPO production, one should determine at least peripheral EPO serum concentrations by immunological methods. Only in cases with elevated EPO serum concentrations does bilateral nephrectomy seem to be indicated.

References

1. Eschbach JW, Funk P, Adamson J, Scribner BH, Finch CA (1967) Eryhtropoiesis in patients with renal failure undergoing chronic dialysis. N Engl J Med 276: 653–658
2. Erslev AJ (1970) Anemia of chronic renal desease. Arch Intern Med 126: 774–780
3. Radtke HW, Claussner A, Erbes PM, Scheuermann EH, Schoeppe W, Koch KM (1979) Serum erythropoietin concentration in chronic renal failure: relationship to degree of anemia and excretory renal function. Blood 54: 877–884
4. Ohno Y, Rege AB, Fisher JW, Barona J (1978) Inhibition of erythroid colony forming cells (CFU-E and BFU-E) in sera of azotemic patients with anemia of renal diseases. J Lab Clin Med 92: 916–923
5. Radtke HW, Rege AB, La Marche MB, Bartos D, Bartos F, Campbell RA, Fisher JW (1981) Identification of spermine as an inhibitor of erythropoiesis in patients with chronic renal failure. J Clin Invest 67: 1623–1629
6. Herforth A, Binswanger U, Largiader F, Frick P (1979) Hohe Haemoglobinkonzentration und hoher Haematokrit bei Traegern von Nierenallotransplantaten. Schweiz Med Wochenschr 109: 1293–1298
7. Dagher FJ, Ramos E, Erslev AJ, Alongi SV, Karmi SA, Caro J (1979) Are the native kidneys responsible for erythrocytosis in renal allografts? Transplantation 28: 496–498
8. Varkarakis MJ, Sampson D, Gerbas JR, Bender MA, Mirand EA, Murphy GP (1971) Polycythemia following renal transplantation unrelated to the allograft. J Surg Oncol 3: 157–161
9. Ianhez LE, Da Fonseca JA, Chocair P, Maspes V, Sabbage E (1977) Polycythemia after kidney transplantation. Influence of the native kidneys on the production of hemoglobin. Urol Int 32: 382–392
10. Wu KK, Gibson TK, Freemann RM (1971) Erythrocytosis after renal transplantation. Its occurrence in two recipients of kidneys from the same cadaveric donor. Arch Intern Med 132: 898–902
11. Tarvazi RC, Froehlich ED, Dustan HP (1966) Hypertension and high hematocrit. Am J Cardiol 18: 855–858
12. Luke RG, Kennedy AC, Stirling WB, McDonald GA (1965) Renal artery stenosis, hypertension and polycythemia. Br Med J 1: 164–166
13. Thevenod F, Radtke HW, Gruetzmacher P, Vincent E, Koch KM, Schoeppe W, Fassbinder W (1983) Deficient feedback regulation of erythropoiesis in kidney transplant patients with polycythemia. Kidney Int 24: 227–232
14. Mirand EA, Murphy GP (1975) Erythropoietin alterations in patients with uremia, renal allograft or without kidneys. JAMA 209: 327–334
15. Eckardt KU, Kurtz A, Hirth P, Scigalla P, Wieczorek L, Bauer C (1988) Evaluation of the stability of human erythropoietin in samples for radioimmunoassay. Klin Wochenschr 66: 241–245
16. Fauser AA, Messner HA (1978) Granuloerythropoietic colonies in human bone marrow, peripheral blood and cord blood. Blood 52: 1243–1248
17. Mollison PL, Engelfriet CP, Contreras M (1979) Antigens on leucocytes, platelets and serum proteins. In: Blood transfusion in clinical medicine, 6th ed Alden, Oxford, pp 690–697
18. Ginn HE (1972) Late medical complications of renal transplantation. Arch Intern Med 116: 6–15
19. Prompt CA, Lee DBN, Upham AT (1977) Medical complications of renal transplantation. II. Non-infectious complications in recipient. Urology 9 [Suppl]: 32–48
20. Chisholm GD (1973) Complications of renal transplantation. Proc R Soc Med 66: 914–918
21. Fisher JW (1972) Erythropoietin: pharmacology, biogenesis and control of production. Pharmacol Rev 24: 459–501
22. Napier JAF, Janowska-Wieczorek A (1981) Erythropoietin measurements in the differential diagnosis of polycythemia. Br J Haematol 48: 393–401

23. Erslev AJ, Caro J, Miller O, Cobbs E (1979) Plasma erythropoietin in polycythemia. Am J Med 66: 243–247
24. Lamperi S, Carozzi S, Manca F, Valente U (1985) Erythropoietin-independent erythropoiesis in polycythemic transplanted patients. Transplant Proc 17: 86–88
25. Shalhoub RJ, Rajan U, Kim VV, Goldwasser E, Kark J, Antoniou LP (1982) Erythrocytosis in patients on long term hemodialysis. Ann Intern Med 97: 686–690
26. Gregory CJ, Eaves AC (1977) Human marrow cells capable of erythropoietic differentiation in vitro: definition of three erythroid colony responses. Blood 49: 855
27. Raghavachar A, Frickhofen N, Arnold R, Schmeiser T, Porzsolt F, Heimpel H (1986) Hematopoietic colony formation after allogeneic bone marrow transplantation: enhancement by cyclosporin A and anti-gamma-(immune) interferon antiserum in vitro. Exp Hematol 14: 621–625
28. Frassoni F, Bacigalupo A, Piaggio G, Podesta M, Repetto M, Marmont AM (1985) Effect of cyclosporin A (CyA) on the in vitro growth of hemopoietic progenitors from normal marrow. Exp Hematol 13: 1084–1088
29. Stockenhuber F, Geissler K, Sunder-Plassmann G, Kurz RW, Steininger R, Muehlbacher F, Hinterberger W, Balcke P: Erythrocytosis in renal graft recipients is not due to elevated erythropoietin serum concentrations. Transplant Proc (in print)

Erythropoietin in the Treatment of Anemia

Recombinant Human Erythropoietin

R. V. BATTERSBY and C. J. HOLLOWAY

Introduction

This paper attempts to review the experimental efforts made to produce recombinant human erythropoietin. In view of its clinical importance, special attention must be paid to its quality in the sense of a functional replacement of the natural hormone. Accordingly, a detailed comparison of the human urinary extracted form with the recombinant product is given. For better understanding, the efforts at cloning and expression of the hormone in various cellular systems are discussed.

The reader should bear in mind that the status of this paper will be that of the date at which the Symposium in Lübeck was held, i.e., June 1988. Due to the enormous commercial potential of erythropoietin, a large number of companies are working on the development of this hormone as a pharmaceutical compound. To date, however, only a product derived from the AMGEN (USA) based procedures has been licensed as a drug.

This paper concentrates, therefore, on the comparison of the erythropoietin extracted from human urine [1] with the recombinant form derived from cell culture production in a line of chinese hamster ovary cells (CHO).

Isolation of the Human Erythropoietin Gene and Expression in CHO Cells

The initial step in the cloning [2] of this gene was the establishment of the complete amino acid sequence after extraction of the hormone from urine. Next, a λ-phage genomic library was screened using 20 bp long DNA probes, which were synthesized according to amino acid sequence data. From a total of approx. 1.5 million phage clones, only a few were selected (after expansion, lysis, hybridization and subsequent autoradiography). The selected clones were then examined for a complete, functional HuEPO gene by expression in 293-cells, an adenovirus-transformed embryonal kidney cell line, followed by radioimmunoassay (RIA) for EPO.

The next step was to generate a cDNA via production and isolation of mRNA. The latter was achieved by insertion of a restriction fragment of the complete gene into a pSV4ST shuttle vector and transfection into COS cells. The vector encompasses an SV 40 origin of replication and thus allows for replication of the vector as an episome in these COS cells. A comparison of the nucleotide sequence derived from the cDNA with the nucleotide sequence established from the original genomic clone and the amino acid sequence clarified the structure of the human EPO gene: The protein region is divided by 4 large introns, is initially translated into a single 193 amino acid peptide which is subsequently modified by limited proteolysis and glycosylation, the sites of which can be predicted according to simple rules.

At this point, it is worth noting that the gene has been expressed in various organisms, including *E. coli* [3], *Saccharomyces cerevisiae* and mammalian cells. It was found, however, that the type of glycosylation was essential for the retainment of full biological activity: The peptide derived from *E. coli* failed in the in vivo bioassay.

The CHO cell line bears a dihydrofolate reductase deletion (DHFR−). The pDSVL vector employed contains (a) a mutant of the bacterial plasmid pBR322, (b) a mouse dihydrofolate reductase minigene, (c) the SV40 origin of replication, promoter region, and the polyadenylation signals, and (d) a *BamH* I restriction endonuclease site. This vector system allows production and selection in bacteria as well as in DHFR(-) cells. Additionally, growing these cells in medium containing methotrexate, an inhibitor of dihydrofolate reductase, will result in an amplification of r-HuEPO production in these cells.

Manufacture of Recombinant Human Erythropoietin

Describing the industrial manufacturing procedures in detail is beyond the scope of this paper, apart from the fact that many of the steps performed are confidential data. Nonetheless, a short description of basic requirements is given.

Initially, from the genetically engineered CHO cells, a master working bank was generated. First, limited dilution cloning was performed in two successive rounds to isolate single cells. Based on RIA, in vivo bioassay, and cell growth characteristics, a limited number of clones were chosen. From these candidate cell banks, one was chosen to be expanded to a master working cell bank at AMGEN, California, which is at present the source of industrial r-HuEPO production.

From this MWCB, one vial is taken to be expanded in cell culture. After an appropriate growth time, the medium is collected and subjected to chromatographic cleaning up to yield the final purified bulk product. The following chapter describes the measures taken to assess the purity and biological potency of this product.

Needless to say, the cell culture systems and the final product are monitored by legal requirements for viral and other contamination by extensive diagnostic procedures.

Structural and Biological Properties of r-HuEPO

Structural Properties

Human erythropoietin is expressed as a single peptide chain consisting of 193 amino acids [4]. During posttranslational modification processes, the 27 amino acid leader sequence *and* the C-terminal arginine in position 166 are cleaved [5], resulting in a peptide of 165 amino acids. Additionally, a total of two disulfide bridges (position 7–161 and 29–33) contributes to the final tertiary structure.

The molecular weight based on the peptide sequence amounts to 18.2 kDa, whereas the hormone entity has a relative molecular weight of approx. 32 kDa (judged by sodium dodecyl sulfate polycrylamide gel electrophoresis, SDS PAGE). The molecular weight determined by sedimentation equilibrium is 30.4 kDa. The discrepancy between the two values is accounted for by extensive glycosylation (ca. 40% of the molecular weight). There are three N-linked (Asp) and one O-linked (Ser) oligosaccharide side chains. The SDS PAGE followed by western blotting with a specific and commercially available monoclonal antibody to EPO [6] is an important biological criterion for the confirmation of the identity of the product.

In isoelectric focusing, various isoforms in the pH-range 4.6–5.1 can be distinguished. These are related to variations in the sialic acid content of the side chains. It is in fact the high sialic acid content which lowers the pI value of the entire hormone considerably because the apparent pI of the unglycosylated peptide (as derived from *E. coli*) is given as 9.2.

Biological Properties

In brief, the biological and immunological properties of u-HuEPO are all shared by r-HuEPO as shown in various test systems:

- In vivo mouse bioassay: This is still the only procedure available that allows for reliable determination of the biological response of this hormone. Two assay models exist; one that measures incorporation of radioactive ^{59}Fe, and another that is based on hematocrit readings.
- In vitro bioassay systems (e.g., cultured bone marrow cells): These do not discriminate effectively between the intact (i.e., fully glycosylated hormone) or deglycosylated forms of the erythropoietin, although they might be favoured from the financial point of view.
- Immunological assays (e.g., RIA). The RIA is used as a rapid means of quantitation. The units of hormone measured will not, however, necessarily reflect a population of biologically intact molecules, and the results obtained will have to be verified by additional measurements.

Comparison of r-HuEPO with u-HuEPO

Chemical Composition

With regard to the amino acid composition after complete hydrolysis, the C-terminal residue, peptide mapping after partial digestion by various proteinases and subsequent high performance liquid chromatography (HPLC) analysis and, finally, the peptide sequence, both proteins must be considered as identical, beyond doubt [4]. Furthermore, the identical positioning of disulfide bonds and the glycosylation sites has been shown.

Physical Characterization

A wide spectrum of analytical methods was applied to obtain relevant data for a comparison of both compounds [7]. The molecular weights obtained after SDS PAGE electrophoresis or gel filtration are very similar for both proteins, even though there are some theoretical problems involved. The former method will be influenced by the anomalous behaviour observed for glycoproteins in general as far as the binding of SDS is concerned, and the latter method actually is based on the Stokes radius rather than molecular weight. On the other hand, sedimentation equilibrium experiments gave a molecular weight for recombinant EPO of 30.4 kDa, which corresponds well with the values achieved by the methods described above.

A comparison on the basis of circular dichroism shows both for the near and distant UV region identical bands within the variability of the method [7]. This is a clear indication for a high degree of similarity in secondary and tertiary structure. Fluorescence spectra and subsequent quenching experiments provide further evidence for structural similarity.

Obvious Structural and Biological Differences

A careful evaluation of electrophoresis experiments revealed differences in values for r-HuEPO and u-HuEPO which must be due to variations in glycosylation. Here, detailed investigations which have just recently been published [8, 9] give an exact description of the oligosaccharide moieties.

The O-linked side chain is only small (four sugar residues) and leaves little room for discussion. The N-linked oligosaccharides, however, seem to play a major role in modulating/maintaining the biological activity of the hormone.

One of the papers cited above [8] has studied the oligosaccharides in great detail after pronase digestion of the peptide moiety. The resulting oligosaccharides were separated by HPLC and subsequently specified by fast atom bombardment mass spectometry (FAB-MS). The results of this work can be summarized as follows:

The N-linked chains consist mainly of tetraantennary oligosaccharides, with minor portions of tri- and biantennary forms, and mostly bearing terminal sialic acid residues. Both erythropoietins are very similar, the major difference lying in the type and degree of sialization. The recombinant hormone contains exclusively NeuAc $\alpha 2 \rightarrow 3$ Gal linkages, whereas, in contrast, the urinary form additionally bears NeuAc $\alpha 2 \rightarrow 6$ Gal linkages (to a degree of approx. 40%). Most of these findings are supported by the opposite approach [9], where the olisaccharide moieties are enzymatically degraded with glycosidases and subjected to further analysis.

Of particular importance is the finding that the recombinant hormone does not contain any new structural elements or differing saccharides, thus any fear of neoantigens which could limit clinical use is eliminated in this system. Therefore, the differences between urinary and recombinant EPO are minimal as far as the structural aspects are concerned.

At this point, however, we still do not fully understand the differences in biological activity between the recombinant and the urinary form. The literature on this particular subject gives specific activities of approx. 70–80 U/μg for the urinary hormone, whereas the recombinant values are above 200 U/μg [5].

The degree and type of glycosylation is, therefore, of special importance for the in vivo biological activity. When the recombinant gene for EPO is expressed in *E. coli,* for example, the correct amino acid sequence is observed with corresponding in vitro biological activity, but the in vivo test (mouse bioassay) shows no response. The biological activity in humans is closely related essentially to a high degree of sialization to avoid rapid hepatic clearance. In a recent paper [10], the expression of EPO (a) under the influence for glycosylation inhibitors and (b) in an insect cell line with reduced glycosylation capacity in comparison to eucaryotic systems is presented. In both cases, r-HuEPO was produced bearing oligosaccharides considerably reduced in size, but still retaining substantial in vivo biological activity. A better understanding of the function of these relevant oligosaccharides will be necessary in the near future to enhance development of biotechnologically derived drug compounds.

Summary

From the widespread efforts to clone and express biologically active erythropoietin suitable for industrial production, only the recombinant hormone from CHO cells has so far been introduced to the market, although there is no doubt about the fact that other companies will follow with similar products. This presentation should satisfy the clinicians interest in the question of biological equivalence. From the data presented, it is fairly safe to say that both proteins considered are very similar and that the existing minimal structural differences do not impair the desired biological efficacy, nor do they bear the risk of provoking an undesirable immunological response due to the presence of neoantigens.

References

1. Lin F-K, Suggs S, Lin C-H et al. (1985) Cloning and expression of the human erythropoietin gene. Proc Natl Acad Sci USA 82, 7580–7584.
2. Lee-Huang S (1984) Cloning and expression of human erythropoietin cDNA in Escherichia coli. Proc Natl Acad Sci USA 81, 2708–2712.
3. Miyake T, Kung CK-H, Goldwasser E (1977) Purification of human erythropoietin. J Biol Chem 252, 5558–5564.
4. Lai PH, Everett R, Wang FF et al. (1986) Structural characterization of human erythropoietin. J Biol Chem 261, 3116–3121
5. Recny JM, Scoble HA, Kim Y (1987) Structural characterization of natural human urinary and recombinant DNA-derived erythropoietin. Identification of des-arginine 166 erythropoietin. J Biol Chem 262, 17156–17163.
6. Sytkowski MA, Fischer JW (1985) Isolation and characterization of an anti-peptide monoclonal antibody to human erythropoietin. J Biol Chem 260, 14727–14731.
7. Davis JM, Arakawa T, Strickland TW et al. (1987) Characterization of recombinant human erythropoietin produced in chinese hamster ovary cells. Biochemistry 26, 2633–2638.
8. Sasaki H, Bothner B, Dell A et al. (1987) Carbohydrate structure of erythropoietin expressed in chinese hamster ovary cells by a human erythropoietin cDNA. J Biol Chem 262, 12059–12076.
9. Takeuchi M, Takasaki S, Miyazaki H, et al. (1988) Comparative study of the asparagine linked sugar chains of human erythropoietins purified from urine and the culture medium of recombinant chinese hamster ovary cells. J Biol Chem 263, 3657–3663.
10. Wojchowski DM, Orkin SH, Sytkowsky AJ (1987) Active human erythropoietin expressed in insect cells using a baculovirus vector: a role for N-linked oligosaccharide, Biochim Biophys Acta 910, 224–232.

Erythropoietin, Blood Viscosity, and Hypertension: Implications for Patients with End-Stage Renal Disease

R. M. SCHAEFER and A. HEIDLAND

Introduction

Recombinant human erythropoietin (r-HuEPO) is a major breakthrough in the management of renal anaemia. This hormone has been shown to be effective in correcting this anaemia in patients maintained by haemodialysis [1–6]. Up to now, patients have been treated for more than 2 years with sustained benefit and without any evidence of loss of efficacy. Nevertheless, the development or aggravation of hypertension in a certain number of patients treated with r-HuEPO has been recognized [1–6] and probably represents the major clinical concern at present. The issue of hypertension is of utmost importance, because renal failure patients display a high rate of cardiovascular morbidity and mortality [7] and because hypertension is a major risk factor for cardiovascular disease [8]. The present review considers our current knowledge of the relationships between hypertension, blood rheology, and haematocrit as well as the implication of hypertension as a risk factor for cardiovascular disease.

Haematocrit, Rheology, and Hypertension

The interrelationship of these three parameters is given in the formula of Poiseuille [9]. Accordingly, vascular resistance will vary directly with blood viscosity, and inversely with the 4th power of vessel radius. Whole blood viscosity is a complex variable depending on haematocrit, plasma viscosity, and red blood cell aggregation and deformability [10]. Since blood behaves as a non-Newtonian fluid, viscosity increases exponentially at low shear rates (microcirculation) due to an increment of red blood cell aggregation. Thus, a combination of high plasma viscosity and elevated red blood cell aggregation can critically limit the microcirculatory flow, while the fluidity in large vessels predominantly depends on the haematocrit [10]. In patients with essential hypertension, both haematocrit and whole blood viscosity have been found to be increased [11]. Leschke et al. [12] made similar observations in patients suffering from renovascular or -parenchymal hypertension. Whatever causes the increase in haematocrit and viscosity, the elevated whole blood viscosity is likely, according to the law of Poiseuille, to contribute to vascular resistance, thereby causing a further increase in blood pressure. Accordingly, Letcher et al. [13] described a direct relationship between blood pressure and viscosity in normal and hypertensive subjects. More recently, the same group documented a relation between whole blood viscosity and left ventricular hypertrophy in hypertensive patients [14]. Intriguingly, this relation was not dependent on blood pressure.

Among patients suffering from end-stage renal disease, those with hypertension tend to have higher haemoglobin levels than normotensive patients [15]. In 1971 Neff and coworkers [16] studied the relation between blood pressure and haematocrit in dialysis patients more thoroughly. Using transfusions of packed red cells, haematocrit levels were increased from 22% to 43%. This caused a fall in cardiac output and an increase in peripheral vascular resistance, which led to an increment in diastolic blood pressure of 20 mmHg. The authors suggested that this was due to an increase in whole blood viscosity, a loss of hypoxic vasodilatation or a combination of both. In 1977, Capelli and Kasparian confirmed those results [17]. Similar observations can be made after successful renal transplantation. Haematocrit levels will rise, causing an increase in vascular resistance and a fall in cardiac output [18]. A certain propensity for hypertension seems to be important in determining whether a given patient will develop frank hypertension following a rise in his haematocrit. Thus, the five out of six patients studied by Neff et al. [16] who became hypertensive after red blood cell transfusions had at least a history of hypertension. Comparable results are available from laboratory studies. Despite a similar degree of anaemia, peripheral vascular resistance was reduced only in spontaneously hypertensive rats, remaining unchanged in normotensive control animals [19].

Taken together, these studies provide evidence for the critical role of hypertension, whether past or present, for the haemodynamic response to changing haematocrit levels. Adaptive structural changes of the arteriolar wall, which occur in hypertension, were suggested by Folkow [20] as one possible explanation.

Erythropoietin, Hypertension, and Haemorheology

With the advent of r-HuEPO effective treatment of renal anaemia has become feasible. Nevertheless, de novo evolution or worsening of hypertension in a considerable proportion of patients treated has been reported by all groups [1–6]. Winearls et al. [1] observed hypertensive encephalopathy in one patient and a grand mal seizure in one patient with severe hypertension. Similar findings were reported by Eschbach and coworkers [2], who described one patient with hypertension and a grand mal seizure. More recently, Schaefer et al. [6] documented hypertension in three out of 15 dialysis patients (20%) treated with r-HuEPO. These authors reported that a haematocrit value of 30% seems to represent a threshold above which severe hypertension occurred and that all three patients threshold above which severe hypertension occurred and that all three patients who became hypertensive had either a history of high blood pressure or were under antihypertensive medication at the start of the trial. Three patients who were suffering from hypotension remained hypotensive during therapy with r-HuEPO. In a larger multi-center study on 150 dialysis patients, which was conducted by Ortho/Cilag [21], 48 patients developed hypertension (32%) during an observation period of 52 weeks. A total of 71 patients (48%) had a history of hypertension. However, only one patient was hypertensive at the onset of the trial. All others were well controlled either with dialysis alone or in combination with antihypertensive drugs. In the majority of patients sufficient blood pressure control during r-HuEPO therapy could be achieved by institution or reinforcement of antihypertensive medication or by a lowering of the haematocrit to under 30%. One patient dropped out due to intractable hypertension. There was only a slight increase in mean predialysis blood pressure from 94.5 mmHg at baseline to 97.1 mmHg after 52 weeks. It was also investigated whether there was any acute effect of intravenous r-HuEPO administration. Blood pressure was monitored immediately before and during the first hour after injection of the hormone. In general, there were no differences of clinical importance. However, a 57-year-old female with arteriosclerosis and a history of hypertension suffered hypertensive encephalopathy 1 h after r-HuEPO administration.

From these early studies it seems that severe hypertension during r-HuEPO therapy might arise in previously hypertensive subjects. Normotensive patients tended to display only a slight and insignificant increase in blood pressure.

From a theoretical point of view blood viscosity should increase with rising haematocrit values in erythropoietin-treated patients. This issue was addressed recently by Schaefer and coworkers [22] who monitored whole blood viscosity and its components during 4 months of r-HuEPO treatment. As could be expected, whole blood viscosity increased with rising haematocrit values both at low (+42%) and high (+33%) shear rates. Since haematocrits were only increased from 24% to 36%, the whole blood viscosity in these patients did not reach those levels which were observed in healthy controls. Intriguingly, these authors documented an elevated plasma viscosity in their group of dialysis patients as compared to healthy volunteers and there was no change in this parameter during r-HuEPO therapy. An elevation in plasma viscosity seems to be prevalent among subjects with chronic renal failure, as similar findings were reported by Leschke et al. [12] in a group of patients with moderate renal failure. The elastic component, as a measure of red cell aggregation, rose considerably with the increment in the haematocrit (+118%) at low shear rates, suggesting that flow conditions in the microcirculation could be influenced unfavourably. Graf and coworkers [23] were able to confirm the findings on blood rheology in r-HuEPO-treated patients on dialysis. When corrected for the rise in haematocrit, however, the increase in whole blood viscosity was appropriate. Nevertheless, the rise in whole blood viscosity will increase peripheral vascular resistance, and it is conceivable that in a certain group of patients cardiac output might fail to decrease adequately and thereby result in arterial hypertension. A second group at risk would be those who display a high plasma viscosity, and it might be sensible to measure fibrinogen levels in these patients before starting with r-HuEPO, as fibrinogen is the main determinant of plasma viscosity.

As a second hypothesis for the rise in blood pressure it has been postulated that the correction of anaemia will abolish hypoxic vasodilatation, which is observed in anaemic patients with [16] and without [24–26] renal failure. Correction of anaemia improves tissue oxygenation [27] and thereby will cause an increment in peripheral vascular resistance, which might contribute to the evolution of high blood pressure.

Finally, a third mechanism has been proposed recently by which r-HuEPO therapy might increase blood pressure [28]. Nitric oxide, a potent natural vasodilatator [29], is produced and secreted together with prostacyclin by endothelial cells [30]. As prostacyclin production is increased in chronic renal failure [31] it could be that nitric oxide is also generated in excess in uremic subjects. On the other hand, haemoglobin is known to rapidly bind nitric oxides [32]. Thus, rising haemoglobin levels during r-HuEPO therapy would trap nitric oxides and would permit unopposed contraction of vascular smooth muscle cells. If this hypothesis were correct, nitroglycerin should be the drug of choice in those patients becoming hypertensive during r-HuEPO treatment, as it mimics the action of endogenous nitric oxides.

Conclusions

Recombinant human erythropoietin is a major breakthrough in the management of patients with end-stage renal disease as it abolishes the need for blood transfusions and improves the quality of life. The rise in haematocrit, however, is associated with an increase in blood viscosity, which might predispose to left ventricular hypertrophy [14], independent of the blood pressure behaviour. Patients with peripheral vascular disease are especially at risk, as flow conditions in the microcirculation are negatively influenced by rising haemotocrit values [22] due to enhanced red cell aggregation. The major clinical problem, however, will be the development or aggravation of hypertension, since high blood pressure is an important risk factor for vascular morbidity and mortality in patients with or without chronic renal failure. Those with a history of hypertension or those who have high blood pressure at the onset of therapy are most likely to develop severe hypertension. If hypertension occurs, several therapeutic options are available, including reduction of the dry weight and institution or reinforcement of conventional antihypertensive therapy. But lowering of haemocrit levels by reduction of the r-HuEPO dose, or even by phlebotomy, might become necessary. In general, the renal anaemia should be corrected gradually within 3–4 months. The target haematocrit should be determined for each patient individually, taking benefits and potential risks into account.

It is known that uraemic patients with relatively high haemotocrits due to polycystic kidney disease do not suffer from an increased cardiovascular or cerebrovascular morbidity. On the contrary cardiac arrest and myocardial infarction are less frequent and the prevalence of cerebrovascular accidents is identical, despite the propensity for cerebral aneurysms, to that in patients with standard primary renal diseases (see the data reported in [33], especially Fig. 15). Based on these observations we think that further long-term clinical trials with r-HuEPO are warranted to exclude the possiblity that improvements in the quality of life of end-stage renal failure patients are associated with an enhanced cardiovascular morbidity and mortality.

Summary

Recombinant human erythropoietin (r-HuEPO) is able to correct anaemia, to abolish the need for further blood transfusions, and to improve the quality of life for patients with end-stage renal disease. On the other hand, the rise in haematocrit will increase blood viscosity and thereby peripheral vascular resistance, which will give rise to frank hypertension in a certain proportion of patients treated with r-HuEPO. As more than 50% of chronic renal failure patients die from cardiovascular and cerebrovascular disease, for which high blood pressure is a recognized risk factor, the development of hypertension is of particular concern. Those patients who are already hypertensive prior to the onset of therapy are most likely to develop severe hypertension. However, given the enormous benefits and the fact that the major risks are now well defined, a careful use of erythropoietin in patients with chronic renal failure seems well justified.

References

1. Winearls CG, Oliver DO, Pippard MJ, Reid C, Downing MR, Cotes PM (1986) Effect of human erythropoietin derived from recombinant DNA on the anaemia of patients maintained by chronic haemodialysis. Lancet 2. 1175–1178
2. Eschbach JW, Egrie JC, Downing MR, Browne JK, Adamson JW (1987) Correction of the renal anemia of end-stage renal disease with recombinant human erythropoietin N Engl J Med 316: 73–78
3. Bommer J, Alexiou C, Müller-Bühl U, Eifert J, Ritz E (1987) Recombinant human erythropoietin therapy in haemodialysis patients – dose determination an clinical experience. Nephrol Dial Transplant 2: 238–242
4. Casati S, Passerini P, Campisi MR, Graziani G, Cesana B, Perisic M, Ponticelli C (1987) Benefits and risks of protracted treatment with human recombinant erythropoietin in patients having haemodialysis. Br Med J 295: 1017–1020
5. Stutz B, Rhyner K, Vögtli J, Binswanger U (1987) Erfolgreiche Behandlung der Anämie bei Hämodialyse-Patienten mit rekombinantem humanem Erythropoietin. Schweiz Med Wochenschr 117: 1397–1402

6. Schaefer RM, Kürner B, Zech M, Krahn R, Heidland A (1988) Therapie der renalen Anämie mit rekombinantem humanem Erythropoietin. Dtsch Med Wochenschr 113: 125–129
7. Raine AEG, Ledingham JGG (1984) Cardiovascular complications after renal transplantation. In: Morris PJ (ed) Kidney transplantation: principles and practice. Grune and Stratton, London, pp 469–489
8. Kannel WB (1977) Importance of hypertension as a major risk factor in cardiovascular disease. In: Genest J, Koiw E, Kuchel O (eds) Hypertension: pathophysiology and treatment. McGraw Hill, New York, pp 888–909
9. Chien S (1977) Blood rheology in hypertension and cardiovascular disease. Cardiovasc Med 2: 356–360
10. Schmid-Schönbein H, Rieger H, Fischer T (1980) Blood fluidity as a consequence of red cell fluidity: flow properties of blood and flow behavior of blood in vascular diseases. Angiology 31: 301–319
11. Tibblin G, Bergentz SE, Bjure J, Wilhelmsen L (1966) Hematocrit, plasma protein, plasma volume, and viscosity in early hypertensive disease. Am Heart J 72: 165–176
12. Leschke M, Motz W, Blanke H, Strauer B (1988) Blood rheology in hypertension and hypertensive heart disease. J Cardiovasc Pharmacol 10 [Suppl 6]: 103–110
13. Letcher RL, Chien S, Pickering TG, Sealey JE, Laragh JH (1981) Direct relationship between blood pressure and blood viscosity in normal and hypertensive subjects. Am J Med 70: 1195–1202
14. Devereux RB, Drayer JIM, Chien S, Pickering TG, Letcher RL, DeYoung JL, Sealey JE, Laragh JH (1984) Whole blood viscosity as a determinant of cardiac hypertrophy in systemic hypertension. Am J Cardiol 54: 592–595
15. Hilden M, Hilden T (1968) Haemoglobin levels and renal function in patients with and without hypertension. Acta Med Scand 183: 183–190
16. Neff MS, Kim KE, Persoff M, Onesti G, Swartz C (1971) Hemodynamics of uremic anemia. Circulation 43: 876–883
17. Capelli JP, Kasparian H (1977) Cardiac work demands and left ventricular function in end-stage renal disease. Ann Intern Med 86: 261–267
18. Kim KE, Bates O, Onesti G, Swartz C (1987) Hemodynamics before and after successful renal transplantation. Abstracts, Xth Int Congress of Nephrol, London, p 286
19. Susic D, Mandal AK, Kentera D (1984) Hemodynamic effects of chronic alteration in hematocrit in spontaneously hypertensive rats. Hypertension 6: 262–266
20. Folkow B (1978) Cardiovascular structural adaptation: its role in the initiation and maintenance of primary hypertension. Clin Sci 55: 3S–22S
21. Sundal E, Bariety J, Bommer J, Canaud B, Danielson B, Kreis H, Lamperi S, Michielsen P, Rhyner K, Ponticelli C, Schaefer RM, Verbeelen D, Zehnder C, Kaeser U (1988) Correction of anaemia of chronic renal failure with recombinant human erythropoietin: results from a multicenter study in 150 haemodialysis-dependent patients. Nephrol Dial Transplant (in press)
22. Schaefer RM, Leschke M, Strauer BE, Heidland A (1988) Blood rheology and hypertension in hemodialysis patients treated with erythropoietin. Am J Nephrol 8: 449–453
23. Mayer G, Steffenelli T, Cada EM, Thum J, Stummvoll HK, Graf H (1988) Blood pressure and erythropoietin (letter). Lancet 1: 351–352
24. Roy SB, Bhatia ML, Mathur VS, Virmani S (1963) Hemodynamic effects of chronic severe anemia. Circulation 28: 346–356
25. Duke M, Herbert VD, Abelmann WH (1964) Hemodynamic effects of blood transfusion in chronic anemia. N Engl J Med 271: 975–980
26. Cropp GJA (1969) Hemodynamic responses to oxygen breathing in children with severe anemia. Circulation 40: 493–499
27. Nonnast-Daniel B, Creutzig A, Kühn K, Reimers E, Bahlmann J, Brunkhorst R, Koch KM (1988) Erythropoietin treatment associated changes of peripheral hemodynamics and tissue oxygenation in renal anemia: early and long-term effects. Abstracts of the XXVth Congress of the European Dialysis and Transplantation Association, pp 213

28. Martin J, Moncada S (1988) Blood pressure, erythropoietin, and nitric oxide. Lancet 1: 644
29. Editorial (1987) EDRF. Lancet 2: 137–138
30. Palmer RMJ, Ferrige AG, Moncada S (1987) Nitric oxide release accounts for the biological activity of endothelium-derived relaxing factor. Nature 327: 525–526
31. Deckmyn H, Proesmans W, Vermyen J (1983) Prostacyclin production by whole blood from children: impairment in the hemolytic uremic syndrome and excessive formation in chronic renal failure. Thromb Res 30: 13–18
32. Martin W, Smith JA, White DG (1986) The mechanism by which haemoglobin inhibits the relaxation of rabbit aorta induced by nitrovasodilatators, nitric oxide or bovine retractor penis inhibitor factor. Br J Pharmacol 89: 562–571
33. Figures from combined report on regular dialysis and transplantation in Europe (1987) XXVth Congress of the European Dialysis and Transplantation Association Fig. 15

Recombinant Human Erythropoietin and *CIS*-Retinoic Acid Therapy of Anemia in Hemodialysis and Peritoneal Dialysis Patients

S. Carozzi, M. G. Nasini, and S. Lamperi

Introduction

The depressed erythropoiesis of uremic anemia is consequent to the reduced proliferation and differentiation of erythroid stem cells, which are due to the deficient production of erythropoietin (EPO) by the kidney [1–3]. This is confirmed by the very recent results concerning recombinant human erythropoietin (rHuEPO) use in uremic dialysis patients, which showed that intravenous administration of this hormone leads to a significant improvement in erythropoiesis [4–6].

Cis-Retinoic acid and its metabolites have been shown to increase the number of burst-forming unit-erythroid (BFU-e) colonies, the more immature erythroid progenitors in vitro in a dose-dependent manner [7]. Thus, besides EPO, also retinoids might be able to correct the defective bone marrow erythroid proliferative activity in uremics.

The aim of this study was, therefore, to evaluate the effects of a *cis*-retinoic acid derivative, etretinate, on the bone marrow and peripheral blood abnormalities in a group of anemic dialysis patients in comparison to a second group of anemic dialysis patients treated with rHuEPO.

Patients and Methods

Of the 25 uremic patients studied, 15 (seven on hemodialysis, HD, for 38.5 ± 11.7 months and eight on continuous ambulatory peritoneal dialysis, CAPD, for 32.8 ± 10.4 months) were treated with etretinate (Tigason, Hoffman-La Roche, Basel, Switzerland) and 10 (on HD for 27.4 ± 7.8 months) were treated with rHuEPO (AMGen, Thousand Oaks, CA; Cilag, Schaffhausen, Switzerland; Ortho Pharmaceutical, Raritan, N.J.).

All patients gave their informed consent to participate in this study. The etretinate group was composed of seven women and eight men (average age 52.3 ± 4.2 years), and the rHuEPO group of five women and five men (average age

54.3 ± 2.5 years). The degree of anemia was comparable for the two groups (hematocrit, Hct: 18.8 ± 5% and 19.1 ± 1.1%; hemoglobin, Hb: 5.9 ± 0.1 and 5.8 ± 0.2 g/dl).

There were also no significant differences between the two groups with regard to nutritional or metabolic state, serum proteins or various other clinical parameters. None of the patients were anephric, had other causes of anemia besides the uremia, had recently been transfused blood, or showed signs of iron overload. The majority had little chance of receiving a renal transplant.

The etretinate or rHuEPO therapy was supplemented with iron or folic acid when necessary.

Etretinate was administered per os at a dosage of 25–50 mg/24 h according to the response and tolerance. It is known, that initially etretinate has a brief half-life (2 h), while after prolonged treatment the half-life increases [8] due to the low elimination capacity. Therefore, during the first phase (12 weeks) etretinate was given twice daily at a dosage of 12.5–25 mg, and during the second phase (16 weeks) as a single daily dose of 25 or 50 mg. The tolerance was good in the majority of cases. In two cases, beginning at the 24th week, an exfoliative dermatitis developed; treatment was suspended and the dermatitis rapidly disappeared.

rHuEPO was given thrice weekly as an intravenous bolus at the end of each dialysis session, in progressively increasing doses according to tolerance, for 32 weeks. The dosages studied ranged from 72 to 554.4 ± 52.6 U/kg b.w./week. The secondary effects consisted of one case of allergic palpebral edema which led to suspension of the drug, and one case of AV fistula clotting problems.

In vitro and in vivo studies of hematologic parameters were performed. In the in vivo studies, Hb levels (g/dl) and reticulocyte, leukocyte, and platelet counts ($10^3/mm^3$) were determined every two weeks in all patients. The Hb levels and reticulocyte counts were assessed by standard methods, while leukocyte and platelet counts were done with a Coulter counter.

In the in vitro studies, the proliferative development of bone marrow burst-forming unit-erythroid (BFU-e) and colony-forming unit-erythroid (CFU-e) was evaluated every 4 weeks in some patients. Bone marrow specimens were obtained by sternal aspiration following local anesthesia, and the culture technique used was the Iscove method [9]. The values were expressed as the number of BFU-e or CFU-e colonies developed per 2×10^5 bone marrow mononuclear cells plated.

Statistics

Results were expressed as mean ± standard error of the mean (SEM). Data were compared using Student's t-test for unpaired observations. Statistical significance between patient groups was assessed by corrected Chi^2 and Fisher's exact tests. Changes between findings before and after etretinate and rHuEPO therapies were analyzed by means of Wilcoxon's matched-pair test. A p value less than 0.05 was considered statistically significant.

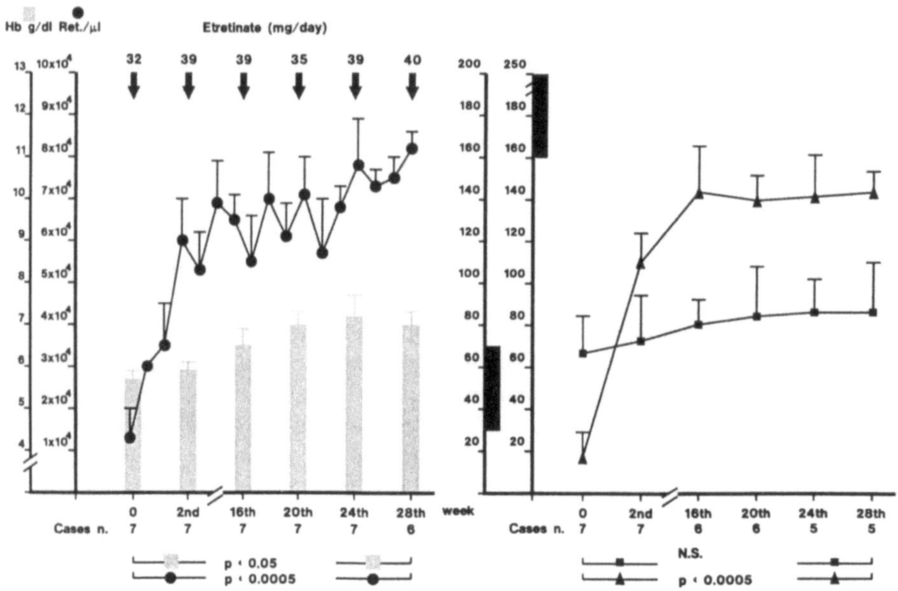

Fig. 1. Per os (p.o.) therapy with etretinate: effects on the hemoglobin levels (*Hb g/dl*), reticulocyte count (*Ret./μl*), and in vitro proliferation of the BFU-e and CFU-e in a group of hemodialysis patients during 28 weeks of drug therapy. The *bars* and the *points* are the means of the Hb levels and the reticulocyte counts respectively. The *triangles* and the *squares* are the BFU-e and CFU-e growths respectively (colonies/2 × 10^5 cells). *Brackets*, standard error of mean; *shaded area*, normal range

Results

Etretinate Therapy

In HD patients, oral treatment with etretinate induced a slow, progressive rise in Hb values, starting from the 16th week and reaching a maximum during the 24th week of therapy (24.1%; $p < 0.05$). A noticeable increase in the reticulocyte count was also seen, beginning in the 2nd week and continuing through the 28th week (485.7%; $p < 0.0005$).

Before etretinate therapy, study of bone marrow erythroid progenitor growth demonstrated that both BFU-e and CFU-e development capacities were significantly decreased as compared with the mean values seen in non-uremic, non-anemic controls (78.2% and 63.8% respectively; $p < 0.0005$). From the 2nd week, treatment induced significant and progressive increases in the number of BFU-e colonies; the highest levels were seen from the 16th to the 28th week, showing a 935.7% rise ($p < 0.0005$). The values reached were, on the average, 190.7% higher than those seen in controls ($p < 0.0005$). Contemporaneously, no significant modification of in vitro CFU-e colony growth was seen (Fig. 1).

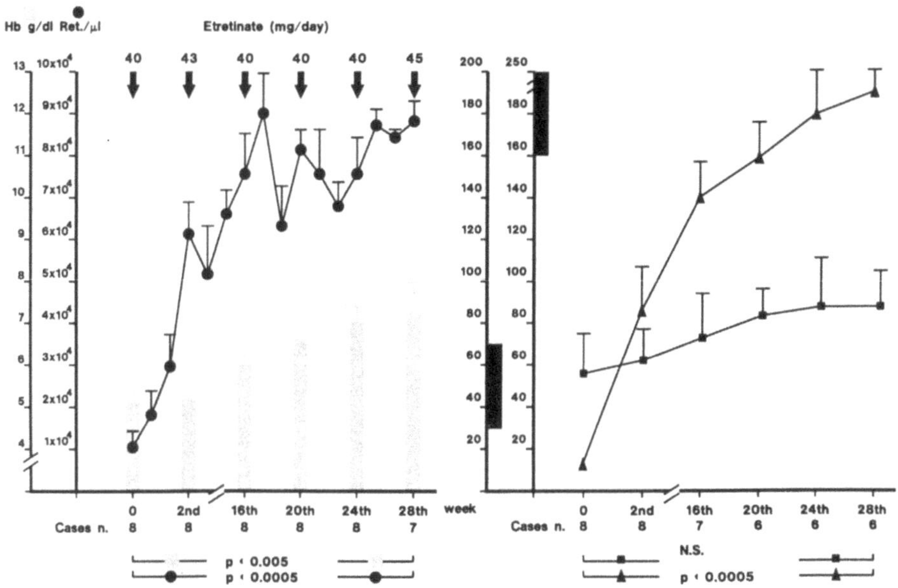

Fig. 2. Per os (p.o.) therapy with etretinate: effects on the hemoglobin levels (*Hb g/dl*), reticulocyte count (*Ret./μl*), and in vitro proliferation of the BFU-e and CFU-e in a group of continuous ambulatory peritoneal dialysis patients during 28 weeks of drug therapy. For explanation of symbols, see Fig. 1

In CAPD patients treated with etretinate, a similar behavior of both peripheral blood and bone marrow hematologic parameters was seen: in the 28th week, Hb values were 44,2% higher than before therapy ($p<0.005$), and there were 1410.2% and 850.5% increases in the reticulocyte count and BFU-e colony number respectively ($p<0.0005$). In these patients, the reticulocyte number as well as the BFU-e growth improvements were significantly more marked at the end of the study period than in the HD patients ($p<0.05$) (Fig. 2).

In both HD and CAPD patients, etretinate therapy caused a progressive rise in the leukocyte count. In HD patients, maximum values were observed in the 28th week (42.6% increase; $p<0.05$), while in CAPD patients the highest levels were observed in the 24th week (51.7%; $p<0.05$). During the entire period of therapy no significant change in the platelet count was seen in either patient group (Tables 1, 2).

rHuEPO Therapy

In HD patients treated for 12 weeks with increasing doses of i. v. rHuEPO (first phase), progressive rises in Hb values were observed from the 2nd week, such that in the 12th week they were 81.2% higher than before therapy ($p < 0.0005$). The

Table 1. Per os therapy with etretinate: effects on the leukocyte and platelet counts in a group of hemodialysis (HD) patients during 32 weeks of drug therapy

	Etretinate therapy							
Weeks	0	4	8	12	16	20	24	28
HD patients (n)	7	7	7	7	7	7	7	6
Leukocytes ($10^3/mm^3$)	6.1 ± 0.4	6.5 ± 0.2	7.1 ± 0.5	7.7 ± 0.1	8.2 ± 0.3*	8.5 ± 0.4*	8.3 ± 0.2*	8.7 ± 0.3*
Platelets ($10^3/mm^3$)	244.1 ± 30.4	256.7 ± 27.5	261.3 ± 34.5	241.5 ± 22.5	260.7 ± 27.3	234.7 ± 30.4	256.7 ± 22.1	231.5 ± 26.1

Data expressed as mean ± SEM
* Significantly different from mean value before therapy ($P < 0.05$)

Table 2. Per os therapy with etretinate: effects on the leukocyte and platelet counts in a group of continuous ambulatory peritoneal dialysis (CAPD) patients during 32 weeks of drug therapy

	Etretinate therapy							
Weeks	0	4	8	12	16	20	24	28
CAPD patients (n)	8	8	8	8	8	8	8	7
Leukocytes ($10^3/mm^3$)	5.8 ± 0.3	6.6 ± 0.4	7.1 ± 0.2	7.7 ± 0.6	7.9 ± 2.0	8.1 ± 0.3*	8.8 ± 2.0*	8.1 ± 0.5*
Platelets ($10^3/mm^3$)	234.5 ± 18.9	248.2 ± 24.3	243.8 ± 28.1	251.7 ± 27.5	265.1 ± 18.5	235.7 ± 18.7	227.7 ± 12.6	231.2 ± 17.9

Data expressed as mean ± SEM
* Significantly different from mean value before therapy ($P < 0.05$)

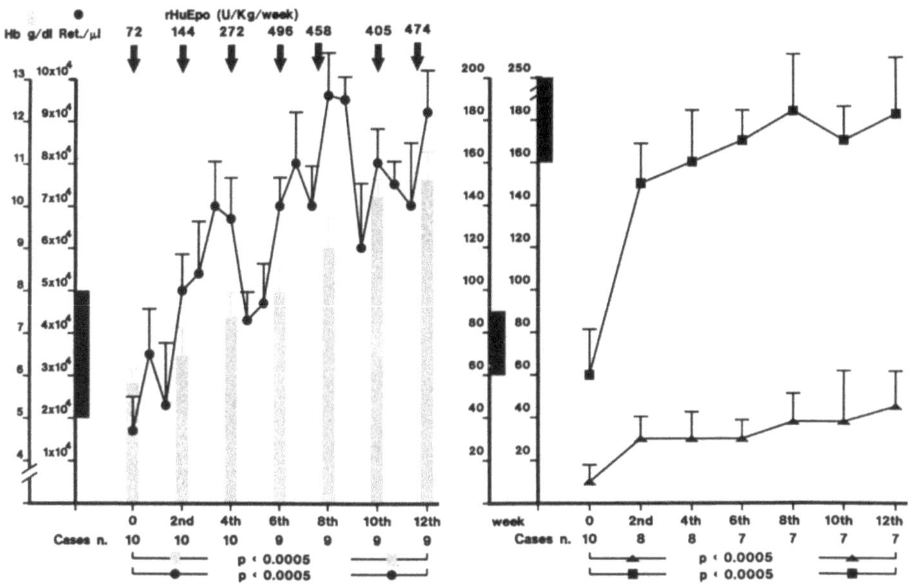

Fig. 3. Intravenous therapy with recombinant human erythropoietin (rHuEPO): effects on the hemoglobin levels (*Hb g/dl*), reticulocyte count (*Ret./μl*), and in vitro proliferation of the BFU-e and CFU-e in a group of hemodialysis patients during the first 12 weeks of hormone therapy. For explanation of symbols, see Fig. 1

reticulocyte count showed similar behavior, reaching maximum values (533.3% increase) in the 8th week ($p < 0.0005$).

In vitro evaluation of bone marrow erythroid proliferative capacity demonstrated a marked improvement of CFU-e colony growth from the 2nd week of therapy. Values detected in the 12th week were 210.1% higher, on the average, than before therapy, and comparable to those seen in non-uremic, non-anemic patients ($p < 0.0005$). Simultaneous evaluation of BFU-e colony growth also revealed a progressive increase (250.7%; $p < 0.0005$). However, values obtained did not in any case reach the normal range (Fig. 3).

During the second phase of therapy, from the 12th to the 32nd week, during which the dose of rHuEPO was equal to the maximum reached at the end of the first phase, the Hb levels remained stationary, while the reticulocyte count decreased, beginning from the 12th week. At the 32nd week (220.5%; $p < 0.0005$), although higher than before therapy ($p < 0.0005$), the reticulocyte count was still 54.2% lower than at the 12th week ($p < 0.0005$).

There was also a slight increase of the BFU-e colonies between the 12th and 16th weeks (27.2%; $p < 0.05$), at which point the levels were still below the normal range and after which they returned to the levels of the 12th week; and a progressive decrease of the CFU-e colonies which, however, remained within the normal range.

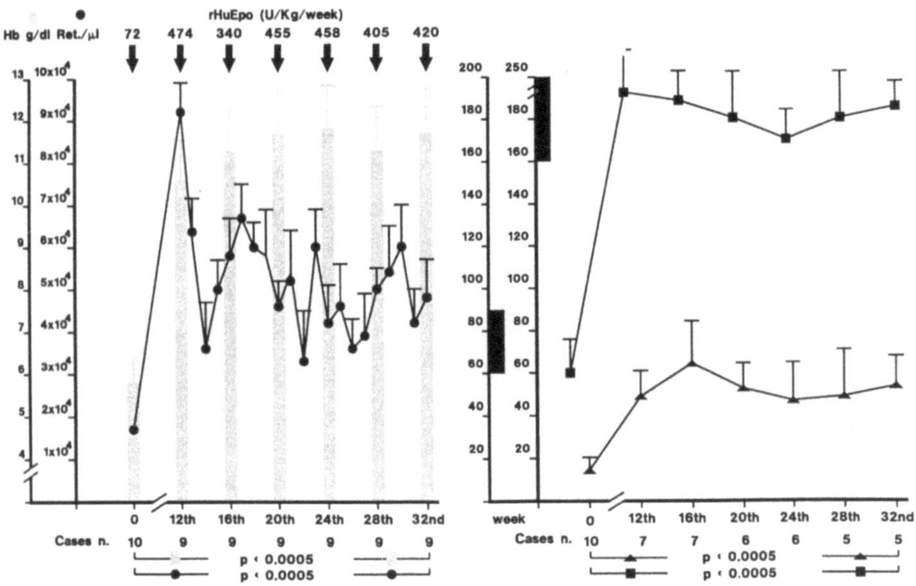

Fig. 4. Intravenous therapy with recombinant human erythropoietin (rHuEPO): effects on the hemoglobin levels (*Hb g/dl*), reticulocyte count (*Ret./µl*), and in vitro proliferation of the BFU-e and CFU-e in a group of hemodialysis patients from the 12th through the 32nd week of hormone therapy. For explanation of symbols, see Fig. 1

Maximum decreases were seen in the 24th week; at that time values were about 25% lower than those seen in the 12th week ($p < 0.05$) (Fig. 4).

Neither in the first nor the second phase did rHuEPO treatment induce significant changes in the leukocyte or platelet count (Table 3).

Discussion

Some data in the literature suggest that retinoids can stimulate the growth and the differentiation of hematopoietic cells. This is shown in vivo by the fact that anemia is one of the clinical manifestations of avitaminosis A [10, 11]. These substances have been shown to act on normal bone marrow stem cells, increasing the proliferation of both the normal progenitors of the granulocyte megakaryocyte (GM) series and the more immature erythroid progenitors. In the presence of retinoids, in fact, the development in vitro of CFU-GM colonies greatly increases; they appear to have a comparable effect on the erythroid progenitors, BFU-e, although there is no complete agreement regarding this [12, 13].

Table 3. Intravenous therapy with recombinant human erythropoietin (rHuEPO): effects on the leukocyte and platelet counts in a group of hemodialysis (HD) patients during 32 weeks of hormone therapy

	rHuEPO therapy				
Weeks	0	4	8	12	16
HD patients (*n*)	10	10	9	9	9
Leukocytes ($10^3/mm^3$)	6.8 ± 0.6	6.1 ± 0.5	7.2 ± 1.1	6.4 ± 0.8	5.7 ± 0.5
Platelets ($10^3/mm^3$)	234.3 ± 29.4	246.2 ± 23.1	243.9 ± 23.5	236.7 ± 24.5	215.1 ± 21.0

	rHuEPO therapy				
Weeks		20	24	28	32
HD patients (*n*)		9	9	9	9
Leukocytes ($10^3/mm^3$)		6.7 ± 0.9	6.0 ± 0.6	6.1 ± 0.3	5.7 ± 0.3
Platelets ($10^3/mm^3$)		241.0 ± 18.5	200.6 ± 20.6	219.8 ± 19.7	233.2 ± 12.6

Data expressed as mean ± SEM

Based on these results, we felt it would be interesting to evaluate the effects of a retinoid, etretinate, on the reduced proliferation of bone marrow erythroid progenitors in uremics with anemia and, consequently, on peripheral hematologic parameters. The results were compared with those obtained in anemic uremics treated with rHuEPO, whose mechanism of action has been clarified by in vitro studies [14, 15] and whose positive effects in vivo on uremic anemia are being documented ever more widely [4, 5].

Our results with etretinate show the possibility of obtaining positive effects on the peripheral hematologic parameters of anemic uremics, consisting of a modest, progressive increase in the levels of Hct, Hb and the leukocyte count, with a significantly greater increase in the number of reticulocytes. In the patients treated with rHuEPO, there were more marked rises in these parameters, except for the leukocyte count, which did not change significantly.

The in vitro effects of etretinate on bone marrow erythroid proliferation also differed from those of rHuEPO. Etretinate stimulated the proliferation and differentiation of the more immature erythroid elements, the BFU-e, which are greatly reduced in anemic uremics, both undergoing HD and CAPD, while in the more mature erythroid precursors, the CFU-e, considered the physiological target of EPO, there was no significant change. This indicates that the mechanism of action of retinoids on bone marrow cells in anemic uremics is different from that of EPO. Retinoids act on the more immature cells and are probably not specific for the erythroid series, but also act on the granulocyte series. On the contrary, the action of EPO is limited to the more mature elements of the erythroid series (CFU-e), extending right through to normoblasts [16].

As the retinoids stimulate only the more immature erythroid progenitors (BFU-e), when EPO is lacking this is not sufficient to affect the peripheral blood hematologic parameters, while EPO leads to the nearly total normalization of the hematologic parameters in anemic uremics. However, our studies have shown that after prolonged therapy, even with relatively high doses of rHuEPO, there tends to be a decrease in the number of CFU-e in vitro, associated with a drop in the reticulocyte count in vivo. This reduction of the effects of rHuEPO is probably due to a deficit of CFU-e, which is secondary to a lack of their precursors, the BFU-e. Since retinoids stimulate the proliferation of BFU-e, their addition to the rHuEPO could help avoid this problem by providing more BFU-e to become CFU-e and be stimulated by EPO.

However, two questions remain unanswered. Why, if etretinate causes such an increase in the reticulocyte count, is there so little change in the red cell count and Hb levels? It is possible that the bone marrow hyperstimulation caused by etretinate determines an abnormal proliferation and differentiation of erythroid precursors and thus the formation of defective reticulocytes. It is also possible that it is only due to the lack of EPO, which is also necessary for the maturation of reticulocytes.

The second question concerns the exact mechanism of action of etretinate on the BFU-e. Does etretinate directly stimulate the proliferation of BFU-e, or does it act indirectly by potentiating the effects of colony-stimulating factor, burst-promoting activity and possibly even EPO? In vitro studies appear to support the indirect mechanism of action [10]. In any case, retinoids could belong to the group of physiological factors which modulate erythropoiesis and become altered during anemia.

In conclusion, our results have shown that etretinate and EPO act at different stages of erythropoiesis. Therefore, the addition of etretinate could potentiate the effects of rHuEPO in the treatment of uremic anemia, as well as permit a reduction of its dosage.

Summary

Erythropoietin (EPO) and *cis*-retinoic acid are able, in vitro, to modulate the proliferative activity of normal early erythroid progenitors, burst-forming unit-erythroid (BFU-e). Thus, to compare the effects of a *cis*-retinoic acid derivative, etretinate, and rHuEPO on the hematologic abnormalities is uremic anemia we studied 25 patients, 15 treated with etretinate and 10 with rHuEPO. The in vivo results showed that etretinate caused a substantial increase in the reticulocyte count, but only a slight rise in hemoglobin levels, while rHuEPO greatly improved both parameters. In vitro studies showed that etretinate stimulates only the more immature erythroid progenitors (BFU-e), while rHuEPO acts mainly on the more mature progenitors, colony-forming unit-erythroid (CFU-e).

While etretinate causes only a slight improvement in uremic anemia, its use in combination with rHuEPO might potentiate the effect of rHuEPO by furnishing a greater number of immature erythroid stem cells to be stimulated to maturity by rHuEPO.

Acknowledgements. The rHuEPO used was kindly gifted by AMGen, Thousand Oaks, California; Cilag, Schaffhausen, Switzerland; and Ortho Pharmaceutical, Raritan, New Jersey.

References

1. Lai PH, Everett R, Wang FF, Azokawa T, Goldwasser E (1986) Structural characterization of human erythropoietin. J Biol Chem 261: 3116–3121
2. Jacobs K, Shoemaker C, Rudersdorf R (1985) Isolation and characterization of genomic and DNA clones of human erythropoietin. Nature 313: 806–810
3. Lin FK, Suggs S, Lin CH (1986) Cloning and expression of the human erythropoietin gene. Proc Natl. Acad Sci USA 82: 7580–7584
4. Winearls CG, Pippard MJ, Downing MR, Oliver DO, Reid C, Cotes PM (1986) Effect of human erythropoietin derived from recombinant DNA on the anemia of patients maintained by chronic hemodialysis. Lancet 22: 1175–1178
5. Eschbach JW, Egrie JC, Downing MR, Browne JK, Adamson JW (1987) Correction of the anemia of the end stage renal disease with recombinant human erythropoietin. N Engl J Med 316: 73–78
6. Dessypris EN, Gleaton JH, Armstrong OL (1987) Effect of human recombinant erythropoietin on human marrow megakaryocyte colony formation in vitro. Br J Haematol 65: 265–269
7. Douer D, Koeffler HP (1982) Retinoic acid enhances growth of human early erythroid progenitor cells in vitro. J Clin Invest 69: 1039–1041
8. Orfanos CE, Ehlert R, Gollnick H (1987) The retinoids. A review of their clinical pharmacology and therapeutic use. Drugs 34: 411–514
9. Iscove NN (1977) The role of the erythropoietin in regulation of population size and cell cycling of early and late erythroid precursors in mouse bone marrow. Cell Tissue Kinet 10: 323–334
10. Doner D, Koeffler HP (1982) Retinoic acid enhances colony stimulating factor induced clonal growth of normal human myeloid progenitor cells in vitro. Exp Cell Res 138: 193–198
11. Kerndrup G, Bendix-Hausen K, Pedersen B, Ellegaard J, Hokland P (1986) Primary myelodysplastic syndrome: treatment of 6 patients with 13-cis retinoic acid. Scand J Haematol 36 (S45): 128–132
12. Koeffler HP (1983) Induction of differentiation of human acute myelogenous leukemia cells: therapeutic implications. Blood 62: 709–721
13. Kerndrup G, Bendix-Hausen K, Pedersen B, Ellegaard J, Hokland P (1987) 13-*cis* retinoic acid treatment of myelodysplastic syndromes. Leuk Res 11: 7–16
14. Fisher JW, Lajtha LG, Buttoo AS, Porteous DD (1965) Direct effects of erythropoietin on the bone marrow of the isolated perfused hind limbs of rabbit. Br J Haematol 11: 342–349
15. Stohlman F Jr (1971) Erythropoietin and erythroid cell kinetics. In: Fisher JW (ed) Kidney hormones. Academic, New York, p 331
16. Erslev AJ (1987) Erythropoietin coming of age. N Engl J Med 316: 101–103

Clinical Effects of Partial Correction of Anemia Using Recombinant Human Erythropoietin on Working Capacity in Dialysis Patients

H. GRAF and G. MAYER

Introduction

Modern dialysis treatment for terminal renal failure enables long-term survival in a majority of patients. In the wake of the early reports of Winearls and Eschbach [1, 2] on the effectiveness of recombinant human erythropoietin (r-HuEpo) in the treatment of renal anemia in patients on chronic hemodialysis, the widespread use of this exciting treatment can be expected shortly. However, because of the high treatment costs, attention is beginning to be focused on the impact that partial correction of anemia will have on dialysis therapy in general. The major issue is certainly the potential improvement of quality of life.

Psychosocial rehabilitation of dialysis patients critically depends on the co-morbidity, which might be in part related to the degree of renal anemia [3, 4]. Quality of life in general includes a number of subjective influences and thus is difficult to assess [3]. Besides the psychological problems of renal replacement therapy, factors like physical fitness are the major obstacles to rehabilitation. It has been shown that physical training can improve exercise capacity in dialysis patients and that this improvement reduces depression and increases performance of pleasant activities [5, 6]. Therefore physical fitness seems to be one key to a better psychosocial rehabilitation in patients on chronic hemodialysis.

Parameters of exercise capacity

One of the most common tests to assess the physical condition is bicycle ergometry with incremental workloads and simultaneous measurement of peripheral oxygen uptake (VO_2) and pulmonary CO_2 delivery (VCO_2). Initially, ventilation, CO_2 production and peripheral oxygen uptake increase linearly with increasing workload. After this initial phase a further increase of workload starts anaerobic glycolysis in order to provide additional energy. Once anaerobic glycolysis has started, lactic acid is produced in increasing quantities. Bicarbonate buffering of lactic acid is followed by an increasing metabolic CO_2 production with an increase in VCO_2.

This point, which can easily be detected by continous measurement of VCO_2 and VO_2, is called the anaerobic threshold (AT) and is the point when there is a nonlinear increase of VCO_2, which no longer parallels the linear increase of VO_2 during graded exercise.

Initially, ventilation increases proportionally with the increased CO_2 output. Tissue and blood pH remain constant only by buffering lactic acid with bicarbonate. CO_2 in the arterial blood remains constant (isocapnic buffering). As a consequence the ventilatory equivalent for CO_2 (which is ventilation/VCO_2) remains constant or decreases slightly, while the ventilatory equivalent for O_2 increases just above the AT. As the work rate is incremented, further metabolic acidosis develops because lactic acid formation overwhelms bicarbonate buffering. Therefore ventilation starts to increase even more rapidly than CO_2 production, causing a decrease in arterial pCO_2 in order to provide respiratory compensation for the exercise-induced lactic acid acidosis. Arterial pCO_2 can be estimated by breath-by-breath determination of end-tidal CO_2 concentration. Therefore the end of isocapnic buffering can be detected by a decrease of end-tidal CO_2 concentration with an increase of end-tidal O_2 concentration.

The importance of the determination of the AT, first described by Wassermann et al. [7] is strengthened by the fact that it is the best determinant available to demarcate the upper limit of work rate which can be maintained for a prolonged period. The higher the work rate above AT, the less its tolerable duration [8, 9]. Beyond AT, at the maximum workload, another key denominator of exercise capacity, namely maximum peripheral oxygen uptake (VO_2 max) can be determined by spiroergometry.

Besides the distinct information on endurance exercise capacity, the determination of AT provides some further advantages. One of the most important is the objectivity of this noninvasive parameter, as it is determined by gas measurement only. VCO_2 max, on the other hand, carries with it the problem of the definition of "maximum", with its high personal input by the performing patient and physician. Therefore the accuracy of VO_2 max critically depends on the patient's compliance [10].

The Role of Hemoglobin

Exercise capacity in general critically depends on the oxygen supply to the cells with increased metabolic activity, and is influenced by several factors. First, the partial pressure of oxygen in the arterial blood is important. In patients on dialysis with normal pulmonary function, pO_2 is within the normal range. Furthermore, the oxygen affinity of hemoglobin affects the diffusion gradient for oxygen from the blood to the muscle mitochondria. In dialysis patients, metabolic acidosis and elevated levels of 2,3-diphosphoglycerate [11] should provide an optimal oxygen availability and thus cannot explain the reduced exercise capacity. One of the most important factors for the low exercise tolerance in patients with end-stage renal disease in general seems to be the lowered hemoglobin concentration due to renal anemia. In a recent study, patients on chronic hemodialysis with a wide range of hemoglobin levels underwent spiroergometry with determination of VO_2 AT and VO_2 max. There was a positive correlation between blood hemoglobin and exercise capacity in the absence of a correlation to any other variable which might influence exercise capacity, like age, sex, control of uremia, body surface area and comorbidity [12].

Anemia per se also influences another key denominator of oxygen supply to the muscle, the cardiac output. As a consequence of anemia, cardiac output at rest is elevated in patients on hemodialysis, mostly due to an elevation of heart rate [13, 14]. Therefore, during exercise the possibility of increasing cardiac output by increasing heart rate is reduced. Several other factors influence the cardiovascular adaption to exercise in anemic patients, e.g. possible cardiodepressive uremic toxins and uremic sympathetic neuropathy, the latter resulting in lower heart rates at maximum workload in dialysis patients than in controls despite an elevated resting heart rate [15].

Summarizing all data available, anemia seems to be the most important pathogenetic factor for the reduced exercise capacity of patients on renal replacement therapy.

Effects of Correction of Anemia

It therefore seemed reasonable to determine exercise capacity in patients on chronic hemodialysis before and after correction of renal anemia by treatment with r-HuEpo.

Nine patients (four male, five female) on chronic intermittent hemodialysis received r-HuEpo. All of them were dependent on regular blood transfusions to maintain hemoglobin levels greater than 6 g/dl. The number of transfusions administered during the time on dialysis (mean 66 ± 29 months) varied from 8 to 242 units (mean 92 units). The hemoglobin levels immediately before the first r-HuEpo administration were < 6 g/dl, and one unit of blood was given before the first r-HuEpo dose.

r-HuEpo was given intravenously 3 times a week at the end of each hemodialysis session, starting at a dose of 100 U/kg body weight (BW). If the hemoglobin values in the 3rd week were below or equal to 5% of the initial value, the r-HuEpo dose was increased by 25 U/kg/dose. When the target hemoglobin value of 10 g/dl was reached, all patients were transfered to maintenance therapy to keep their hemoglobin levels above 10 g/dl. The maintenance dose was equal to the last dose administered, but was given only twice a week [16]. Eight patients underwent spiroergometry immediately before r-HuEpo therapy, when target hemoglobin was reached and after 3 months of r-HuEpo treatment. One patient was not able to take part in the test because of gonarthrosis.

Exercise testing was performed on a bicycle ergometer starting at a workload of 25 W with increments of 10 W per minute until subjective exercise maximum was reached. All determinations of gas concentrations and volumes were done on line during exercise testing using a microprocessor controlled system (Sensormedics Horizon System VI, Sensormedics, Anaheim, California) [17].

As criterion for exercise capacity, oxygen consumption at subjective exercise maximum (VO_2 max) and at anaerobic threshold (VO_2 AT) was determined.

Dialysis time was calculated using a urea kinetic modelling system in order to keep predialysis BUN levels below 80 mg/dl, which resulted in a comparable degree of uremia in all patients [18].

Anaerobic threshold, a good parameter of endurance work ability, was determined as described by Wasserman et al. as a nonlinear increase in CO_2 production and an increase in end-tidal O_2 without a corresponding change in end-tidal CO_2 [7]. As described elsewhere [19], partial correction of renal anemia immediately leads to better exercise capacity. A significant increase in VO_2 AT was seen immediately after r-HuEPO treatment [13.9 ± 2.0 vs 18.5 ± 3.7 ml O_2/kg BW, $p = 0.01$, Fig. 1), as was an increase in VO_2 max (17.2 ± 4.2 vs 23.1 ± 7.2 ml O_2/kg BW, $p = 0.01$, Fig. 2). This is in accordance with the increment of watt levels reached at AT and VO_2 max (Figs. 3, 4).

After maintenance therapy for 3 months, mean hemoglobin level remained the same (target Hb 10.6 ± 1.0 g/dl vs 10.7 ± 0.8 g/dl after 3 months, $p = 0.9$), as did mean VO_2 at subjective exhaustion (23.1 ± 7.2 vs 22.7 ± 5.2 ml O_2/kg, $p = 0.7$, Fig. 2). However, VO_2 AT increased (18.5 ± 3.7 vs 20.4 ± 3.3 ml O_2/kg BW, $p = 0.004$, Fig. 1), although hemoglobin levels and peripheral oxygen availability was unchanged [20].

Because until recently the clinical significance of lowered blood hemoglobin values in patients with end-stage renal disease was not clearly evaluated, the benefit of even partial correction of anemia by r-HuEpo has been a matter of discussion – all the more since several adverse treatment effects have been reported, placing the cost-benefit relationship in question.

The rise in blood pressure noted by many authors [1, 2, 16] seems to be due to the rise in blood viscosity as well as to the rise in systemic peripheral resistance [21]. The latter might be a consequence of the diminished hypoxic vasodilatation after improvement of oxygen availability [22].

Furthermore, a decrease in plasma volume such as accompanies the rise of hematocrit could decrease solute removal during hemodialysis and therefore could contribute to the increase in predialysis concentrations of BUN, creatinine and potassium as noted by Eschbach [2].

The increased incidence of fistula clotting as reported by Eschbach and by Winearls [1, 2] mostly seems to be due to the rise in blood viscosity. The same finding has been reported in patients with polycystic kidney disease, who primarily differ from other dialysis patients with respect to their hematocrit values [23]. However, life expectancy has been shown to be better in these patients despite their higher risk for infection and hemorrhage when compared to patients with other underlying renal diseases [24].

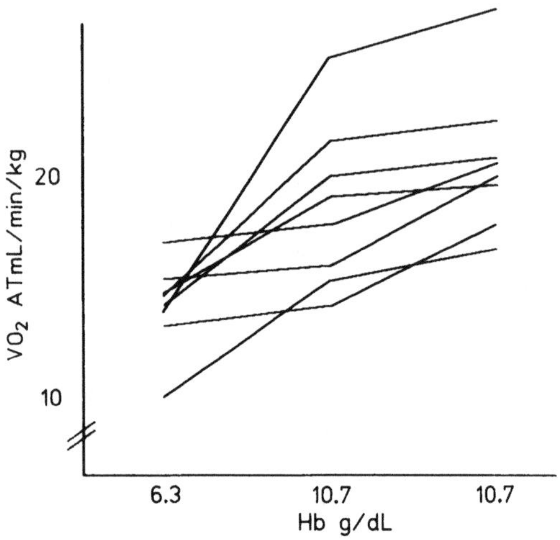

Fig. 1. Oxygen consumption (ml/min/kg) at the anaerobic threshold (*VO_2AT*) before r-HuEpo treatment and after 12 and 24 weeks

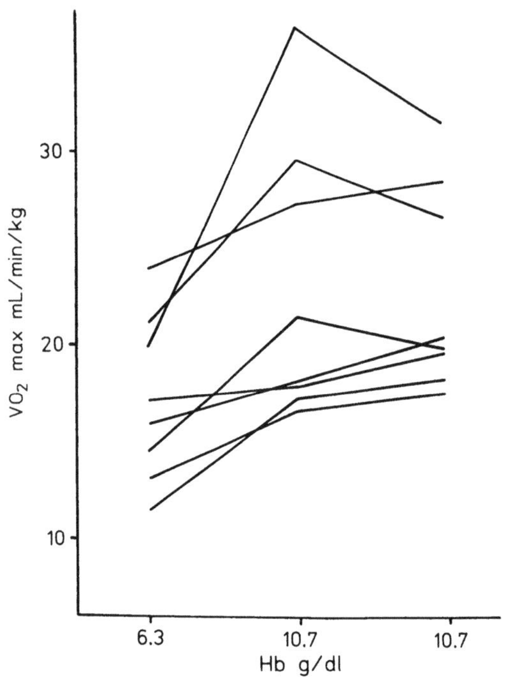

Fig. 2. Maximum oxygen consumption (ml/min/kg) at subjective exhaustion (*$VO_2 max$*) before r-HuEpo treatment and after 12 and 24 weeks

It has recently been shown that a linear correlation exists between blood hemoglobin values and working capacity, and thus social rehabilitation, in patients on chronic hemodialysis [12]. Exercise capacity as measured by VO_2 AT and VO_2 max was improved significantly after successful treatment of renal anemia by

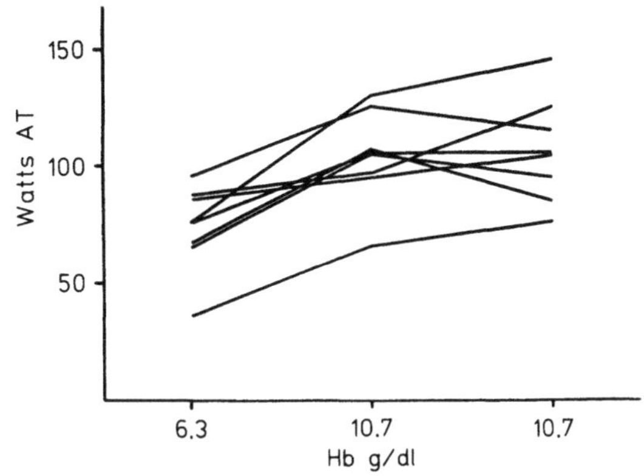

Fig. 3. Workload level (watts) reached at anaerobic threshold (*AT*) before r-HuEpo treatment and after 12 and 24 weeks

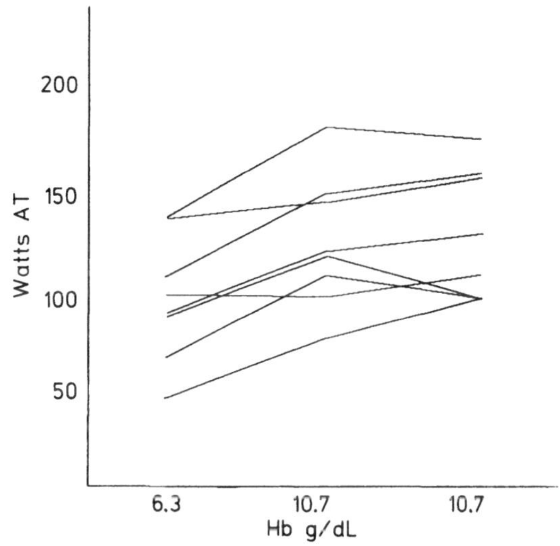

Fig. 4. Maximum workload level (watts) reached before r-HuEpo treatment and after 12 and 24 weeks

r-HuEPO. As expected, working capacity before treatment is less than 50% of the expected values for individuals of the same age and sex. Also, AT is reached at very low work rates. The mean value of 13.9 ml/min/kg means an AT that does not even allow the patient to walk faster than 5 km/h over a longer period. As reported earlier, after partial correction of anemia both VO_2 max and VO_2 AT increased significantly even after a relatively short treatment period [19]. In this respect our data confirm the importance of blood oxygen-carrying capacity for exercise tolerance. Some of these results, however, appear to question oxygen availability as the only cause for exercise limitation.

In patients with long-term but constant-degree anemia there was a linear correlation between exercise capacity and blood hemoglobin values [12]. In our patients, however, there was no correlation between the rise of blood hemoglobin and the improved exercise capacity as measured by VO_2 AT and VO_2 max during the study period. Despite constant hemoglobin values there was a further increase of VO_2 max and VO_2 AT – only the latter significant however – after a prolonged treatment period of 6 months. One possible explanation for these two facts could be that besides oxygen availability, oxygen utilization is of outstanding importance.

The skeletal muscle may be considered a machine that is fueled by the chemical energy of ingested carbohydrates and lipids. This chemical energy is primarily converted to adenosine triphosphate. Various enzymes are needed to gain this high-energy phosphate from free fatty acids and glycogen. Chronic hypoxia per se has been shown to alter muscle enzyme contents and therefore further blunts additional energy supply. West et al. found that lowlanders exposed to high altitude over more than 10 weeks undergo adaptive changes in their aerobic and anaerobic performance [25]. After 5–8 weeks they found a 10%–15% decrease of muscle mass, a 35% decrease of muscle proteins and a 45% reduction of succinate dehydrogenase activity. This resulted in a decrease of both VO_2 max and VO_2 AT. This reduction in energy-providing capacity seems to be a time-related phenomenon, as short-term hypoxia does not influence muscle enzymes [26].

According to West et al., key glycolytic enzymes such as pyruvate kinase, glucose-6-phosphate dehydrogenase and phosphofructokinase have been shown to be reduced in patients with renal anemia [27, 28]. It might well be that the pathogenesis of the reduced working capacity in patients on renal replacement therapy is multifactorial.

Lowered arterial oxygen content per se decreases peripheral oxygen availability and thus working capacity. Furthermore, long-term hypoxia might induce muscular changes. After partial correction of anemia, exercise capacity initially increases rapidly due to the improvement in oxygen availability. Under sustained improvement of oxygen supply muscular enzyme content returns to normal, thus enabling a further improvement of working ability.

In summary, our results show that renal anemia, an almost invariable feature of patients on renal replacement therapy, strongly impairs working capacity in these patients. Even partial correction of anemia by r-HuEpo treatment results in a rapid increase of working capacity, due to the increased oxygen availability, and therefore improves the physical and psychological state [29] of patients on chronic hemodialysis. Long-term treatment with r-HuEPO increases working capacity even further despite constant hemoglobin levels, perhaps because of adaptive changes in muscular enzyme content.

References

1. Winearls CG, Oliver DO, Pippard MJ, Reid C, Downing MR, Cotes PM (1986) Effect of human erythropoietin derived from recombinant DNA on the anaemia of patients maintained by chronic haemodialysis. Lancet II: 1175–1177
2. Eschbach JW, Egrie JC, Downing MR, Browne JK, Adamson JW (1987) Correction of the anaemia of end stage renal disease with recombinant human erythropoietin. N Engl J Med 316: 73–78
3. Evans RW, Manninen DL, Garrison LP, Hart LG, Blagg CR, Gutman RA, Hull AR, Lowrie EG (1985) The quality of life of patients with end stage renal disease. N Engl J Med 312: 553–559
4. Brynger H, Brunner FP, Chantler C, Doncker Wolke RA, Jakobs C, Kramer P, Selwood NH, Wing AJ (1980) Combined report on regular dialysis and transplantation in Europe. Proc Eur Dial Transpl Assoc 17: 3–10
5. Goldberg AP, Geltman EM, Hagberg JM, Gavin JR, Delmez ME, Carney RM, Naumowicz A, Oldfield M, Harter H (1983) The therapeutic benefits of exercise training for haemodialysis patients. Kidney Int 16: s303–s309
6. Carney RM, Templeton B, Hong BA, Harter HR, Hagberg JM, Schechtman KB, Goldberg Ap (1987) Exercise training reduces depression and increases the performance of pleasant activities in haemodialysis patients. Nephron 47: 194–198
7. Wassermann K, Whipp BS, Koyal SN, Beaver WL (1973) Anaerobic threshold and respiratory gas exchange during exercise. J Appl Physiol 35: 236–243
8. Wassermann K (1984) The anaerobic threshold measurement to evalute exercise performance. Am Rev Respir Dis [Suppl] 129: 535–540
9. Kumagai S, Tanaka K, Matsura Y, Matzuzaka A, Hirakoba K, Asano K (1982) Relationship of the anaerobic threshold with the 5 km, 10 km and 10 miles races. Eur J Appl Physiol 49: 13–23
10. Löllgen H (1986) Kardiopulmonale Funktionsdiagnostik, 4th edn. Edition Ciba
11. Lichtman M, Miller DR (1970) Erythrocyte glycolysis, 2,3-diphosphoglycerate and adenosine triphosphate concentration in uremic subjects: relationship to extracellular phosphate concentration. J Lab Clin Med 76: 267–279
12. Mayer G, Thum J, Graf H (1989) Anaemia and reduced exercise capacity in patients on chronic haemodialysis. Clin Sci 76: 265–268
13. Neff MS, Kim KE, Persoff M, Onesti G, Swartz C (1971) Hemodynamics in anaemic patients. Circulation 18: 876–883
14. Mayer G, Steffenelli TH, Thum J, Cada EM, Stummvoll HK, Graf H (1988) Haemodynamic parameters and blood viscosity in the pathogenesis of erythropoietin treatment related hypertension. Nephrol Dial Transpl (abstr) 3: 499
15. Painter P, Messer-Rehak D, Hanson P, Zimmermann SW, Glass NR (1986) Exercise capacity in haemodialysis, CAPD, and renal transplant recipients. Nephron 42: 47–51
16. Graf H, Mayer G, Cada EM, Thum J, Stummvoll HK (1987) Wirksamkeit von rekombinantem humanem Erythropoietin in der Behandlung der transfusionsabhängigen Anämie chronischer Dialysepatienten. Wien Klin Wochenschr 24: 855–859
17. Jones NL (1984) Evaluation of a microprocessor controlled exercise testing system. J Appl Physiol 57: 1312–1318
18. Graf H, Irschik H, Kovarik J, Stummvoll HK (1986) A new algorithm for individual dialysis prescription. Med Prog Technol 11: 191–196
19. Mayer G, Thum J, Cada EM, Graf H (1988) Working capacity is increased following r-HuEpo treatment. Kidney Int 34: 525–528
20. Mayer G, Thum J, Cada EM, Stummvoll HK, Graf H (1988) Verhalten der aeroben und anaeroben Leistungsfähigkeit chronischer Haemodialyse Patienten unter einer Dauertherapie mit rekombinantem humanem Erythropoietin. Nephron 51 (Suppl): 34–38
21. Mayer G, Stefenelli T, Cada EM, Thum J, Stummvoll HK, Graf H (1988) Blood pressure and erythropoietin. Lancet I: 351–352

22. Cropp GJA (1969) Hemodynamic responses to oxygen breathing in children with severe anemia. Circulation 15: 493–500
23. Chester AC, Argy WP, Rakowski TA, Schreiner GE (1978) Polycystic kidney disease and chronic haemodialysis. Clin Nephrol 10: 129
24. Brenner BM, Rector FC (eds) (1986) The kidney. Saunders, Philadelphia
25. West JB (1986) Lactate during exercise at extreme altitude. Fed Proc 45: 2953–2957
26. Young AS, Evens WS, Fisher EC, Sharp RL, Costill DL, Maher JT (1984) Skeletal muscle metabolism of sea level natives following short term high altitude residence. Eur J Appl Physiol 52: 463–466
27. Metcoff J, Lindeman R, Baxter D, Pederson J (1978) Cellular metabolism in uremia. Am J Clin Nutr 30: 1627–1637
28. Nakad T, Fujiwara S, Isoda K, Miyahara T (1982) Impaired lactate production by skeletal muscle with anaerobic exercise in patients with chronic renal failure. Nephron 31: 111–115
29. Graf H, Koniecna T, Sachs E, Cada EM, Mayer G (1988) Psychological effects of correction of anemia by recombinant human erythropoietin in patients on chronic hemodialysis. Clin Res 36: 519 A

In Vitro and In Vivo Regulation of Erythropoiesis

A. GANSER and D. HOELZER

Erythropoiesis involves a cascade of differentiation steps that are driven by a variety of glycoproteins, including interleukin-1 alpha (IL-1α) and interleukin-3 (IL-3), the colony-stimulating factors (CSF) and erythropoietin (Epo) [8, 13, 62]. While the CSF induce the proliferation and differentiation of the pluripotent and committed progenitor cells [8], maturation of the late erythroid progenitors and erythroid precursors is mainly controlled by Epo [25].

The analysis of the early events in erythropoiesis, before the cells become identifiable as proerythroblasts, can only be accomplished by functional assays, i.e. by the capacity of these cells to form colonies in vitro in semisolid media [13, 32, 45, 61, 62]. Using these culture methods it has been possible to identify several erythropoietic compartments which despite representing a continuum can be distinguished by the morphological appearance in situ, i.e. by the size and cellular composition of the colonies formed by the respective progenitor cells. The multipotent progenitors CFU-GEMM (colony-forming unit – granulocyte, erythrocyte, macrophage, megakaryocyte) [16] still possess the capacity to differentiate into the various lineages in vitro upon stimulation by IL-3, granulocyte-macrophage CSF (GM-CSF), G-CSF, M-CSF and Epo [18, 31, 47, 48, 58].

The erythroid progenitor cells have been classified into three distinct compartments [12, 27, 43]. Primitive burst-forming units-erythroid (BFU-E) give rise to larger colonies of more than eight clusters, while the mature BFU-E are composed of three to eight clusters. The most mature erythoid progenitor cells, preceding the hemoglobin-synthezising cells by only two or three cell generations, have been termed CFU-E and usually give rise in vitro to small discrete clusters, each consisting of 8–50+ tightly associated erythroblasts [32]. These different progenitors differ by cell size, density, growth factor requirements, sensitivity to erythropoietin and cell cycle status [54]. Cell cycle analysis with a high dose of tritiated thymidine revealed a progressive increase in cycling activity (for review see [13]). While only 10% –30% of CFU-GEMM and primitive BFU-E are in S-phase, this percentage rises to 40% –50% for mature BFU-E and to 80% for the cells in the CFU-E compartment, i.e. virtually all CFU-E are actively progressing through cell cycle in normal man [64].

Factors Influencing Early Erythropoiesis

Both CFU-GEMM and primitive BFU-E require the presence of factors released from activated lymphocytes and monocytes for survival in vitro [16, 23]. Recombinant DNA technology and the cloning of CSF has allowed the identification of IL-1α [30], IL-3 [24, 44, 46, 59] and GM-CSF [35, 46, 48, 49) as factors possessing burst-promoting activity (BPA) for primitive BFU-E and multipotential stimulating activity for CFU-GEMM, while G-CSF and M-CSF do not seem to have an activity on these progenitors in vitro on their own [46]. A further factor supporting early erythropoiesis is erythroid potentiating activity (EPA) [17]. The capacity of IL-3 to stimulate CFU-GEMM and BFU-E exceeds that of GM-CSF and is not further enhanced by the addition of GM-CSF, indicating that GM-CSF-responsive CFU-GEMM and BFU-E are a subpopulation of the IL-3-responsive progenitors [55]. When several factors are added simultaneously in vitro, G-CSF and GM-CSF synergize with IL-3 in stimulating the growth of CFU-GEMM, but not of BFU-E, which is already maximally stimulated by IL-3. Synergism in the stimulation of CFU-GEMM is similarly seen between IL-1a and GM-CSF, while both cytokines act additively on the growth of BFU-E. While IL-3, GM-CSF, and G-CSF are required to maintain multipotent progenitor cells in culture, Epo does not act at the multipotent progenitor cell level but is only required for the terminal differentiation to hemoglobin-synthezising cells to allow their recognition in vitro [17, 51].

It has been proposed by Van Zant and Goldwasser [68, 69] that CSF and Epo compete for bone marrow progenitor cells with regard to stem cell commitment along the erythroid or myeloid cell lineages. However, Metcalf and Johnson failed to observe this competition between Epo and GM-CSF in vitro [47]. Furthermore, Epo levels have no effect on mouse stem cells in vivo [6], supporting the presently most widely accepted opinion that Epo has no effect on the survival and proliferation of the early erythroid progenitors CFU-GEMM and BFU-E. The in vivo administration of IL-3 to mice, however, results in the stimulation of early and late erythropoiesis with an increase in the total number of CFU-GEMM, BFU-E, and CFU-E [37]. The cycling rate of bone marrow-derived CFU-GEMM as well as of primitive and mature BFU-E is equally increased after in vivo treatment with IL-3. Synergism has also been observed for in vivo combinations of IL-3 and M-CSF, IL-3 and GM-CSF, and GM-CSF and M-CSF. Synergism with regard to the number of hemopoietic progenitor cells in the bone marrow is observed as well, although it is less pronounced [5].

Erythropoietin

The recombinant cloning of murine and human Epo has allowed analysis of effect of the purified molecule both in vitro and in vivo [13, 34, 42]. The activity of Epo is restricted to the later stages in the erythroid lineage [26, 29]. Primitive BFU-E and CFU-GEMM apparently are insensitive to Epo when using highly enriched progenitor cell populations and need Epo only for terminal differentiation in vitro [35]. The mature BFU-E which are the presumed immediate precursors of the CFU-E are partly regulated by Epo. In vitro, these mature BFU-E do not require BPA but fail to survive even in the presence of BPA when addition of Epo is delayed for more than 48 h [60]. To achieve a comparable cloning efficiency, mature BFU-E require a higher concentration of Epo than CFU-E, even when all other known growth factors are present in optimal amounts. The CFU-E are absolutely dependent on the presence of Epo for proliferation [36]. Using pure populations of CFU-E, Nijhoff et al. [53] could show that in mice normal bone marrow CFU-E were very sensitive to even a 5-h deprivation of Epo. The same authors also presented evidence that Epo causes an increase in globin messenger RNA in CFU-E.

Epo acts through binding at specific binding sites which have been identified on normal CFU-E [57]. Binding of Epo is not competitively inhibited by other growth factors, i.e. insulin-like growth factors I and II (IGF-I, IGF-II) and epidermal growth factor, or by insulin or transferrin [57, 63]. Similarly, the other hemopoietic cytokines like IL-3, GM-CSF, G-CSF and interleukin-2 (IL-2) do not interfere with the binding of Epo, as demonstrated in murine cell lines [57]. However, IL-3 can down-regulate the Epo-receptor [63] as it does the receptors for GM-CSF, G-CSF, and M-CSF [65]. The reason why IL-3 should down-modulate Epo receptors on erythroblasts is not clear, but this action could be part of a mechanism for coupling cell growth and differentiation [65]. Thereby, Epo appears to be integrated into the hierarchy of the hemopoietic growth factors necessary to finely tune hematopoiesis [8].

Morphological studies have revealed an effect of Epo on the release of reticulocytes into the bone marrow sinuses [56]. In vivo administration of Epo to experimental animals leads to a withdrawal of perisinal adventitial cells from the parenchymal side of the endothelial cells, resulting in an increased outflow of reticulocytes [56].

Besides its effect on erythropoiesis, Epo has been implicated in the in vitro proliferation and differentiation of megakaryocytic progenitor cells CFU-Mk (CFU-megakaryocyte) [10, 11, 38, 50, 66]. However, the stimulatory activity of Epo on CFU-Mk could not be reproduced using serum-depleted assay systems, indicating that Epo might affect human megakaryopoiesis only by interacting with other hemopoietic factors present in serum, plasma, or conditioned media [7]. Epo seems to have an effect on the later stages of megakaryocytic maturation, where it increases the DNA content of the megakaryocytes [33] and their serotonin content [52]. The apparent lack of an effect on early stages of megakaryopoiesis is also supported by the observation that Epo does not induce megakaryocytic differentiation of the pluripotent CFU-GEMM [19].

Other Factors Influencing BFU-E and CFU-E

IGF-I [1, 40, 41], IGF-II [9], and insulin [9] all potentiate the proliferation of both BFU-E and CFU-E at concentrations reached in human serum. Further factors comprise human growth factor, androgens, thyroid hormone, β-adrenergic agents (for review see [62]) as well as cholesterol contained in the low-density lipoprotein fraction [39].

Effect of Recombinant Human CSF and Erythropoietin In Vivo

Recombinant human Epo (rhEpo), GM-CSF, G-CSF, and IL-3 are now being studied in clinical trials. While the results of bone marrow cultures in patients treated with G-CSF [3] or GM-CSF [4, 22] did not demonstrate any stimulatory effect on the erythroid progenitors BFU-E, in contrast to in vitro findings, the phase I trial with recombinant IL-3 has only recently been started and no data are yet available.

In contrast, phase I and II clinical trials of rhEpo in patients with anemia of end-stage renal disease have been going on for several years, allowing researchers to study the role of erythropoietin in the regulation of erythropoiesis in vivo [2, 15, 28, 67, 70]. The clinical results without exception demonstrate that the anemia is reversed in these patients by treatment with Epo.

The target cells in vivo have been analyzed but the action of Epo on the progenitor cells in vivo is still incompletely understood [20, 21]. When the concentration of circulating hemopoietic progenitor cells was measured in patients undergoing therapy with Epo for anemia of chronic renal failure at dosages between 40 U/kg and 120 U/kg, a significant increase was found not only of the number of BFU-E but also of the number of CFU-GEMM (Fig. 1). This increase mainly occurred during the first week of therapy and was independent of the amount of Epo given to the patients. In addition, the size of the erythroid bursts taken from the blood of the patients after the first week of treatment was considerably larger than at the time points before or afterwards, supporting the hypothesis that at least a subset of BFU-E is activated in vivo by treatment with Epo. The increase in the number of hemopoietic progenitor cells was followed by an increase in the hemoglobin levels and the corrected reticulocyte counts (Tables 1 and 2).

The underlying physiological mechanisms responsible for these changes could include direct and indirect stimulation of a subset of the erythroid progenitor cells BFU-E by Epo [35, 58, 60], modulation of the Epo receptor [57, 63] and a shift of Epo-responsive non-circulating BFU-E into the peripheral blood as described for the release of reticulocytes in animal models [56]. Since pluripotent CFU-GEMM do not directly respond to Epo [51], the observed increase in the number of circulating CFU-GEMM probably is an indirect effect, or simply due to a release of sessile progenitor cells into the circulation.

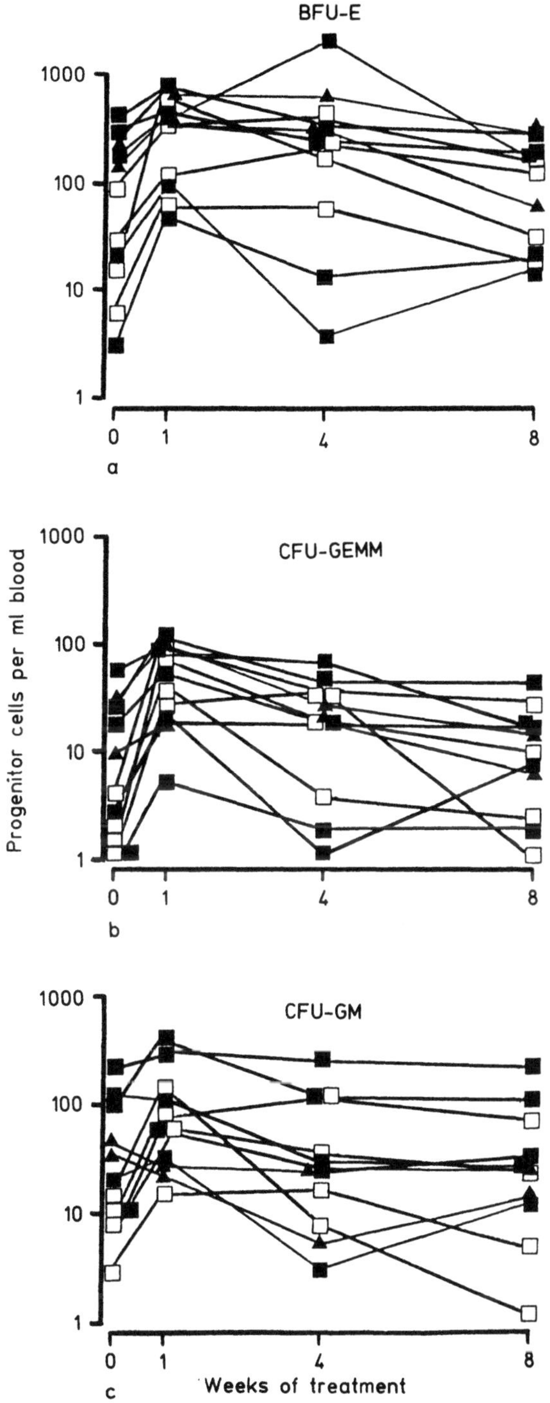

Fig. 1 a–c. Effect of treatment with rhEpo on the concentration of circulating **a** erythroid progenitors BFU-E, **b** multipotential hemopoietic progenitors CFU-GEMM, and **c** granulocyte-macrophage progenitors CFU-GM in patients with anemia of chronic renal failure (■, 40 U/kg; ▲, 80 U/kg; □, 120 U/kg)

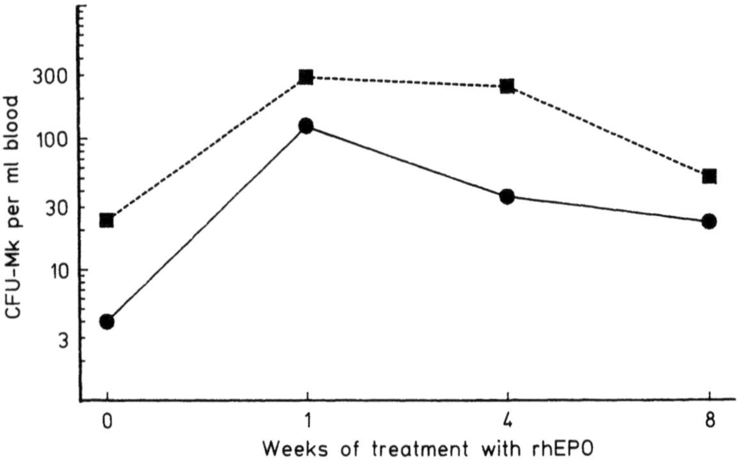

Fig. 2. Effect of treatment with rhEpo on circulating CFU-MK in two patients treated with rhEpo. •, M.L., 40 U EPO/kg; ▪, U.N., 80 U EPO/kg

In agreement with data obtained with murine and human cells in vitro [10, 11], treatment with Epo may increase the number of circulating CFU-Mk (Fig. 2). In addition to its effect at later stages, where it increases the DNA content of the megakaryocytes [33], Epo therefore seems to influence megakaryopoiesis at the progenitor cell level in vivo, probably in combination with other factors [7, 50] and either by stimulation of proliferation or by a shift into the blood. While early results did not demonstrate any effect of treatment with Epo on the platelet counts of the patients [15, 66], more recent trials clearly revealed a dose-related increase in mean platelet numbers [28].

The number of circulating CFU-GM is not influenced by therapy with Epo, excluding the proposed diversion of multipotent progenitor cells along the erythroid differentiation pathway with a subsequent decrease in the number of granulocytic monocytic colonies [68].

In conclusion, in vitro colony assays combined with refined biochemical analyses have provided major insights into the processes which occur during erythropoietic proliferation and differentiation. Various cytokines are involved in the regulation of this pathway, of which only the stimulatory could be mentioned within the framework of this review. Treatment of patients with Epo most certainly results in a whole cascade of interacting events which not only render the analysis more complicated but also permit the study of the relevance of in vitro findings for clinical applications. Therefore, it is important to clarify these mechanisms in order to define the potential role of Epo in the treatment of other disorders of erythropoiesis.

Table 1. Hemoglobin levels (g/dl) after treatment with rhEpo (x ± SEM)

rhEpo	Weeks of treatment with rhEpo				
(U/kg)	− 1	0	+ 1	+ 4	+ 8
40 (n = 5)	7.7 ± 0.3	7.5 ± 0.3	7.5 ± 0.3	8.4 ± 0.4*	9.4 ± 0.6*
80 – 120 (n = 6)	7.6 ± 0.4	7.2 ± 0.4	7.5 ± 0.4	9.0 ± 0.4*	9.7 ± 0.4*

* $P < 0.05$

Table 2. Change in the corrected reticulocyte counts (mean % ± SEM)

rhEpo	Weeks of treatment with rhEpo		
(U/kg)	+ 1	+ 4	+ 8
40 (n = 5)	0.71 ± 0.36*	0.18 ± 0.22	0.13 ± 0.39
80 – 120 (n = 6)	0.27 ± 0.26	0.52 ± 0.25*	0.13 ± 0.31

* $P < 0.05$

References

1. Akahane K, Tojo A, Urabe A, Takaku F (1987) Pure erythropoietic colony and burst formations in serum-free culture and their enhancement by insulin-like growth factor I. Exp Hematol 15: 797–802
2. Bommer J, Müller-Bühl E, Ritz E, Eifert J (1987) Recombinant human erythropoietin in anaemic patients on haemodialysis. Lancet I: 392
3. Bronchud MH, Potter MR, Morgenstern G, Blasco MJ, Scarffe JH, Thatcher N, Crowther D, Souza LM, Alton NK, Testa NG, Dexter TM (1988) In vitro and in vivo analysis of the effects of recombinant human granulocyte colony-stimulating factor in patients. Br J Cancer 58: 64–69
4. Broxmeyer HE, Cooper S, Williams DE, Hangoc G, Gutterman JU, Vadhan-Raj S (1988) Growth characteristics of marrow hematopoietic progenitor/precursor cells from patients on a phase I clinical trial with purified human granulocyte-macrophage colony-stimulating factor. Exp Hematol 16: 594–602
5. Broxmeyer HE, Williams DE, Hangoc G, Cooper S, Gillis S, Shadduck RK, Bicknell DC (1987) Synergistic myelopoietic actions in vivo after administration to mice of combinations of purified natural murine colony-stimulating factor 1, recombinant murine interleukin 3, and recombinant murine granulocyte/macrophage colony-stimulating factor. Proc Natl Acad Sci USA 84: 3871–3875
6. Bruce WR, McCulloch EA (1964) The effect of erythropoietic stimulation on the hemopoietic colony-forming cells of mice. Blood 23: 216–232
7. Bruno E, Bridell R, Hoffman R (1988) Effect of recombinant and purified hematopoietic growth factors on megakaryocytic colony formation. Exp Hematol 16: 371–377

8. Clark SC, Kamen R (1987) The human hematopoietic colony-stimulating factors. Science 236: 1229–1237
9. Dainiak N, Kreczko S (1985) Interactions of insulin, insulinlike growth factor II, and platelet derived growth factor in erythropoietic culture. J Clin Invest 76: 1237–1242
10. Dessypris EN, Gleaton JH, Armstrong OL (1987) Effect of human recombinant erythropoietin on human marrow megakaryocyte colony formation in vitro. Br J Haematol 65: 265–269
11. Dukes PP, Egrie JC, Strickland TW, Browne JK, Lin FK (1986) Megakaryocyte colony stimulating activity of recombinant human and monkey erythropoietin. In: Levine RF, Williams N, Levine J, Evatt BL (eds) Megakaryocyte development and function. Liss, New York, 105–109
12. Eaves CJ, Eaves AC (1978) Erythropoietin dose-response curves for three classes of erythroid progenitors in normal human marrow and in patients with polycythemia vera. Blood 52: 1196–1210
13. Eaves CJ, Eaves AC (1985) Erythropoiesis. In: Golde DW, Takaku F (eds) Hematopoietic stem cells. Dekker, New York, pp 19–43
14. Egrie JC, Strickland TW, Lane J, Aoki K, Cohen AM, Smalling R, Trail G, Lin FK, Browne JK, Hines DK (1986) Characterization and biological effects of recombinant human erythropoietin. Immunobiology 172: 213–224
15. Eschbach JW, Egrie JC, Downing MR, Browne JK, Adamson JW (1987) Correction of anemia of end-stage renal disease with recombinant human erythropoietin: results of a combined phase I and II clinical trial. N Engl J Med 316: 73–78
16. Fauser AA, Messner HA (1978) Granuloerythropoietic colonies in human bone marrow, peripheral blood and cord blood. Blood 52: 1243–1248
17. Gasson JC, Golde DW, Kaufman SE, Westbrook CA, Hewick RM, Kaufman RJ, Wong GG, Temple PA, Leary AC, Brown EL, Orr EC, Clark SC (1985) Molecular characterization and expression of the gene encoding human erythroid-potentiating activity. Nature 315: 768–771
18. Ganser A, Elstner E, Hoelzer D (1985) Megakaryocytic cells in mixed haemopoietic colonies (CFU-GEMM) from the peripheral blood of normal individuals. Br J Haematol 59: 627–633
19. Ganser A, Völkers B, Scigalla P, Hoelzer D (1988) Effect of human recombinant erythropoietin on human progenitor cells in vitro. Klin Wochenschr 66: 236–240
20. Ganser A, Bergmann M, Völkers B, Grützmacher P, Hoelzer D (1988) In vitro and in vivo effects of recombinant human erythropoietin on human hemopoietic progenitor cells. Contrib Nephrol 66: 123–130
21. Ganser A, Bergmann M, Völkers B, Grützmacher P, Scigalla P, Hoelzer D (1989) In vivo effects of recombinant human erythropoietin on circulating human hemopoietic progenitor cells. Exp Hematol (in press)
22. Ganser A, Völkers B, Greher J, Ottmann OG, Walther F, Becher R, Bergmann L, Schulz G, Hoelzer D (1989) Recombinant human granulocyte-macrophage colony-stimulating factor in patients with myelodysplastic syndromes – a phase I/II trial. Blood 73: 31–37
23. Golde DW, Quan SG, Cline MJ (1978) Human T lymphocyte cell line producing colony-stimulating activity. Blood 52: 1068–1072
24. Goodman JW, Hall EA, Miller KL, Shinpock SG (1985) Interleukin 3 promotes erythroid burst formation in „serum-free" cultures without detectable erythropoietin. Proc Natl. Acad Sci USA 82: 3291–3295
25. Graber SE, Krantz SB (1978) Erythropoietin and the control of red blood cell production. Annu Rev Med 29: 51–66
26. Gregory CJ (1976) Erythropoietin sensitivity as a differentiation marker in the hemopoietic system. Studies of three erythropoietic colony responses in culture. J Cell Physiol 89: 289–302
27. Gregory CJ, Eaves AC (1978) Three stages of erythropoietic progenitor cell differentiation distinguished by a number of physical and biological properties. Blood 51: 527–537
28. Grützmacher P, Bergmann M, Weinreich T, Nattermann U, Reimers E, Pollock M (1988) Beneficial and adverse effects of correction of anemia by recombinant human erythropoietin in patients on maintenance hemodialysis. Contrib Nephrol 66: 104–113

29. Hara H, Ogawa M (1977) Erythropoietic precursors in mice under erythropoietic stimulation and suppression. Exp Hematol 5: 141–148
30. Hoang T, Haman A, Goncalves O, Letendre F, Mathieu M, Wong GG, Clark SC (1988) Interleukin 1 enhances growth factor-dependent proliferation of the clonogenic cells in acute myeloblastic leukemia and of normal human primitive hemopoietic precursors. J Exp Med 168: 463–474
31. Ikebuchi K, Clark SC, Ihle JN, Souza LM, Ogawa M (1988) Granulocyte colony-stimulating factor enhances interleukin 3-dependent proliferation of multipotential hemopoietic progenitors. Proc Natl Acad Sci USA 85: 3445–3449
32. Iscove NN, Guilbert LJ, Weyman C (1980) Complete replacement of serum in primary cultures of erythropoietin-dependent red cell precursors (CFU-E) by albumin, transferrin, iron, unsaturated fatty acid, lecithin and cholesterol. Exp Cell Res 126: 121–126
33. Ishibashi T, Koziol JA, Burstein SA (1987) Human recombinant erythropoietin promotes differentiation of murine megakaryocytes in vitro. J Clin Invest 79: 286–289
34. Jacobs K, Shoemaker C, Rudersdorf R, Neill SD, Kaufman RJ, Mufson A, Seehra J, Jones SS, Hewick R, Fritsch EF, Kawakita M, Shimizu T, Miyake T (1985) Isolation and characterization of genome and cDNA clones of human erythropoietin. Nature 313: 306–310
35. Kannourakis G, Johnson GR (1988) Fractionation of subsets of BFU-E from normal human bone marrow: responsiveness to erythropoietin, human placental-conditioned medium, or granulocyte-macrophage colony-stimulating factor. Blood 71: 758–765
36. Kennedy WL, Alpen EL, Garcia JF (1980) Regulation of red blood cell production by erythropoietin: normal mouse bone marrow in vitro. Exp Hematol 8: 1114–1122
37. Kindler V, Thorens B, De Kossodo S, Allet B, Eliason JF, Thatcher D, Farber N, Vassalli P (1986) Stimulation of hematopoiesis in vivo by recombinant bacterial murine interleukin 3. Proc Natl Acad Sci USA 83: 1001–1005
38. Koike K, Shimizu T, Miyake T, Ihle JN, Ogawa M (1986) Hemopoietic colony formation by mouse spleen cells in serum-free culture supported by purified erythropoietin and/or interleukin 3. In: Levine RF, Williams N, Levine J, Evatt BL (eds) Megakaryocyte development and function. Liss, New York, pp 33–49
39. Konwalinka G, Breier C, Geissler D, Peschel C, Wiedermann CJ, Patsch J, Braunsteiner H (1988) Proliferation and differentiation of human erythropoiesis in vitro: effect of different human lipoprotein species. Exp Hematol 16: 125–130
40. Kurtz A, Jelkmann W, Bauer C (1982) A new candidate for the regulation of erythropoiesis: IGF I. FEBS Lett 149: 105–108
41. Kurtz A, Härtl W, Jelkmann W, Zapf J, Bauer C (1985) Activity in fetal bovine serum that stimulates erythroid colony formation in fetal mouse livers is insulinlike growth factor I. J Clin Invest 76: 1643–1648
42. Lin FK, Suggs S, Lin CH et al. (1985) Cloning and expression of the human erythropoietin gene. Proc Natl Acad Sci USA 82: 7580–7584
43. Linch DC, Lipton JM, Nathan DG (1985) Identification of three accessory cell populations in human bone marrow with erythroid burst-promoting properties. J Clin Invest 75: 1278–1284
44. Lopez A, To L, Yang YC, Gamble J, Shannon M, Burns G, Dyson P, Juttner C, Clark S, Vadas M (1987) Stimulation of proliferation, differentiation and function of human cells by primate interleukin 3. Proc Natl Acad Sci USA 84: 2761–2765
45. Messner HA, Jamal N, Izaguirre C (1982) The growth of large megakaryocyte colonies from human bone marrow. J Cell Physiol [Suppl] 1: 45–51
46. Messner HA, Yamasaki K, Jamal N, Minden MM, Yang YC, Wong GG, Clark SC (1987) Growth of human hemopoietic colonies in response to recombinant gibbon interleukin 3: comparison with human recombinant granulocyte and granulocyte-macrographe colony-stimulating factor. Proc Natl Acad Sci USA 84: 6765–6769
47. Metcalf D, Johnson GR (1979) Interactions between purified GM-CSF, erythropoietin and spleen conditioned medium on hemopoietic colony formation in vitro. J Cell Physiol 99: 159–174

48. Metcalf D, Johnson GR, Burgess AW (1980) Direct stimulation by purified GM-CSF of the proliferation of multipotential and erythroid precursor cells. Blood 55: 138–147
49. Migliaccio AR, Bruno M, Migliaccio G (1987) Evidence for direct action of human biosynthetic (recombinant) GM-CSF on erythroid progenitors in serum-free culture. Blood 70–1867–1871
50. Mizoguchi H, Fujiwara Y, Sasaki R, Chiba H (1986) The effect of interleukin-3 and erythropoietin on murine megakaryocyte colony formation. In: Levine RF, Williams N, Levine J, Evatt BL (eds) Megakaryocyte development and function. Liss, New York, pp 111–115
51. Monette FC, Sigounas G (1988) Growth of murine multipotent stem cells in a simple "serum-free" culture system: role of interleukin-3, erythropoietin, and hemin. Exp Hematol 16: 250
52. Nagasawa T, Neichi T, Satoh K, Nakazawa M, Abe T (1988) In vitro regulatory mechanisms for cytoplasmic maturation of murine megakaryocytes derived from colony-forming units (CFU-M). Exp Hematol 16: 667–673
53. Nijhof W, Wierenga PK, Sahr K, Beru N, Goldwasser E (1987) Induction of globin mRNA transcription by erythropoietin in differentiating erythroid precursor cells. Exp Hematol 15: 779–784
54. Ogawa M, MacEachern MD, Avila L (1977) Human marrow erythropoiesis in culture: II. Heterogeneity in the morphology, time course of colony-formation, and sedimentation velocities of the colony-forming cells. Am J Hematol 3: 29–36
55. Ottmann OG, Abboud M, Welte K, Souza LM, Pelus LM (1989) Stimulation of human hematopoietic progenitor cell proliferation and differentiation by recombinant human interleukin 3. Exp Hematol (in press)
56. Papayannopoulou T, Finch CA (1972) On the in vitro action of erythropoietin. J Clin Invest 51: 1179–1185
57. Sawada K, Krantz SB, Kans JS, Dessypris EN, Sawyer S, Glick AD, Civin CI (1987) Purification of human erythroid colony-forming units and demonstration of specific binding of erythropoietin. J Clin Invest 80: 357–366
58. Sieff CA, Emerson SG, Mufson A, Gesner TG, Nathan DG (1986) Dependence of highly enriched human bone marrow progenitors on hemopoietic growth factors and their response to recombinant erythropoietin. J Clin Invest 77: 74–81
59. Sieff CA, Niemeyer CM, Nathan DG, Ekern SC, Bieber FR, Yang YC, Wong GG, Clark SC (1987) Stimulation of human hematopoietic colony formation by recombinant gibbon multi-colony-stimulating factor or interleukin 3. J Clin Invest 80– 818
60. Strife A, Lambek C, Wisniewski D, Gulati S, Gasson JC, Golde DW, Welte K, Gabrilove JL, Clarkson B (1987) Activities of four purified growth factors on highly enriched human hematopoietic progenitor cells. Blood 69: 1508–1523
61. Tepperman AD, Curtis JE, McCulloch EA (1974) Erythropoietic colonies in cultures of human marrow. Blood 44: 659–669
62. Testa NG (1979) Erythroid progenitor cells: their relevance for the study of hematological disease. Clin Hematol 8: 311–333
63. Tsao JC, Tojo A, Fukamachi H, Kitamura T, Saito T, Urabe A, Takaku F (1988) Expression of the functional erythropoietin receptors on interleukin 3-dependent cell lines. J Immunol 140: 89–93
64. Udupa KB, Reissman Kr (1978) Cell kinetics of erythroid colony-forming cells (CFU-e) studied by hydroxyurea injections and sedimentation velocity profile. Exp Hematol 6: 398–404
65. Walker F, Nicola NA, Metcalf D, Burgess AW (1985) Hierarchical down-modulation of hemopoietic growth factor receptors. Cell 43: 269–276
66. Williams N, Jackson H, Iscove NN, Dukes PP (1984) The role of erythropoietin, thrombopoietic stimulating factor, and myeloid colony-stimulating factors on murine megakaryocyte colony formation. Exp Hematol 12: 734–740
67. Winearls CG, Oliver DO, Pippard MJ, Reid C, Downing MR, Cotes PM (1986) Effect of human erythropoietin derived from recombinant DNA on the anaemia of patients maintained by chronic haemodialysis. Lancet II: 1175–1178

68. Van Zant G, Goldwasser E (1977) Simultaneous effects of erythropoietin and colony-stimulating factor on bone marrow cells. Science 198: 733–735
69. Van Zant G, Goldwasser E (1979) Competition between erythropoietin and colony stimulating factor for target cells in mouse bone marrow. Blood 53: 946–965
70. Zins B, Drüeke T, Zingraffe J, Bererhi L, Kreis H, Naret C, Delors S, Castaigne JP, Peterlongo F, Casadevall N, Varet B (1986) Erythropoietin treatment in anaemic patients on haemodialysis. Lancet II: 1329

Sachverzeichnis

MIX
Papier aus verantwortungsvollen Quellen
Paper from responsible sources
FSC® C105338

If you have any concerns about our products,
you can contact us on
ProductSafety@springernature.com

In case Publisher is established outside the EU,
the EU authorized representative is:
Springer Nature Customer Service Center GmbH
Europaplatz 3, 69115 Heidelberg, Germany

Printed by Libri Plureos GmbH
in Hamburg, Germany